Ahmed N. Al-Jamal

Artificial Intelligence

Ahmed N. Al-Jamal

Artificial Intelligence

The development of artificial intelligence

Noor Publishing

Cover image: www.ingimage.com

Publisher:
Noor Publishing
is a trademark of
Dodo Books Indian Ocean Ltd. and OmniScriptum S.R.L publishing group

120 High Road, East Finchley, London, N2 9ED, United Kingdom
Str. Armeneasca 28/1, office 1, Chisinau MD-2012, Republic of Moldova, Europe
Managing Directors: Ieva Konstantinova, Victoria Ursu
info@omniscriptum.com

Printed at: see last page
ISBN: 978-620-9-42688-9

ARTIFICIAL INTELLIGENCE

DR. AHMED NAJI AL-JAMAL

بسم الله الرحمن الرحيم

- <u>فَافْتَحْ بَيْنِي وَبَيْنَهُمْ فَتْحًا وَنَجِّنِي وَمَنْ مَعِيَ مِنَ الْمُؤْمِنِينَ</u> **﴿118﴾**
- <u>فَأَنْجَيْنَاهُ وَمَنْ مَعَهُ فِي الْفُلْكِ الْمَشْحُونِ</u> **﴿119﴾**

صدق الله العلي العظيم

سورة الشعراء

الإهداء

الى:

الذين يصنعون فجراً جديداً في فضاء العلم والمعرفة التماساً لغدٍ منشود

اهدي جهدي المتواضع

المؤلف

INTRODUCTION

Artificial intelligence is a branch of computer science. Many authors define it as: “the study and design of intelligent agents.” An intelligent agent is a system that perceives its environment and takes actions that increase its chances of success in achieving its mission or the mission of its team.

Artificial intelligence (AI) is a field of computer science dedicated to solving cognitive problems typically associated with human intelligence, such as learning, creativity, and image recognition. Modern organizations collect vast amounts of data from a variety of sources, such as smart sensors, human-generated content, monitoring tools, and system logs. The goal of AI is to create self-learning systems that extract meaning from data. AI can then apply that knowledge to solve novel problems in human-like ways. For example, AI can respond meaningfully to human conversations, generate authentic images and text, and make decisions based on real-time data inputs. Your organization can integrate AI capabilities into your applications to improve your business processes, enhance customer experiences, and accelerate innovation. AI has the potential to deliver a range of benefits to a variety of industries.

By overcoming complex problems, increasing business efficiency, making smarter decisions, and automating business processes, AI has a wide range of uses. While not an exhaustive list, here are a few examples that highlight the various use cases for AI. These include intelligent document processing, application performance monitoring, predictive maintenance, medical research, and business analytics.

Artificial intelligence relies on facial, voice and shape recognition systems, which has made its use widespread in daily life and in many different fields. It is used in industry, automation, expert systems, medicine, biology, education and even games.

In the field of medicine, there are programs to diagnose diseases based on known symptoms using logic, probabilities and reasoning so that the automated expert has skills close to the human element.

In the field of language, intelligent systems have been used in linguistic proofreading, morphology, grammar and addressing people, but although machine translation has made great progress at the present time, it has not reached the same quality provided by a human translator, and most programs have failed to achieve this due to their inability to understand the context of speech.

Artificial intelligence is a term used to describe the capabilities of machines and programs that mimic the mental capabilities of humans, such as learning, inference, and reaction to situations that were not programmed into the machine. It is also the name of an academic field concerned with how to create computers and programs capable of adopting intelligent behavior.

It is a prominent feature of the modern era, developed by humans to serve them in accomplishing their tasks with great accuracy, high speed, and solid reliability.

This achievement was accompanied by economic challenges that caused a huge gap in the distribution of wealth between developed and developing countries, and between individuals themselves in the same country, and it became a major threat to a number of jobs.

The term artificial intelligence was introduced by the American computer scientist John McCarthy (1927-2011), who coined it in 1956, the year in which a scientific conference was held at Dartmouth College in the United States to refer to the research being conducted at the time on the possibility of designing an intelligent machine capable of imitating and simulating human work.

Reinforcement learning with human feedback (RLHF) is an additional layer of training that uses human feedback to help ChatGPT learn to follow directions and generate responses that are satisfactory to humans.

OpenAI is best known for its DALL E model, a deep learning model that generates images from textual instructions called prompts.

ChatGPT is a large language model (LLM). LLMs are trained on massive amounts of data to accurately predict the next word in a sentence. It has been found that as the amount of data increases, language models can do more.

The LLM predicts the next word in a sequence of words in a sentence and the following sentences — sort of like autocomplete, but on a mind-bending scale.

This ability allows them to write entire paragraphs and pages of content. But the LLM is limited because it doesn't always understand exactly what a human wants.

There are three factors driving the development of AI across industries.

- Availability of high-performance computing capabilities at an affordable price. The abundance of computing power in the cloud has made it easy to access high-performance computing capabilities at an affordable price. Prior to this development, the only computing environments available for AI were non-cloud-based and expensive.
- Existence of large amounts of data available for learning. AI needs to learn from a lot of data to make accurate predictions. The ease of labeling data and the storage and processing of structured and unstructured data allows for more training and building of algorithms.
- Applied AI provides a competitive advantage. Companies are increasingly realizing the competitive advantage of applying AI insights to business objectives and making them a business priority. For example, targeted recommendations provided by AI can help make better decisions faster. Many of the features and capabilities of AI can also lead to lower costs, reduce risk, accelerate time to market, and more.

The emergence of AI-powered solutions and tools means that more businesses can leverage AI at a lower cost and in less time. Off-the-shelf AI refers to solutions, tools, and software that either have AI capabilities built in or automate algorithmic decision-making. Off-the-shelf AI includes self-healing databases and pre built models for image recognition and analytics.

Author

CONTENTS

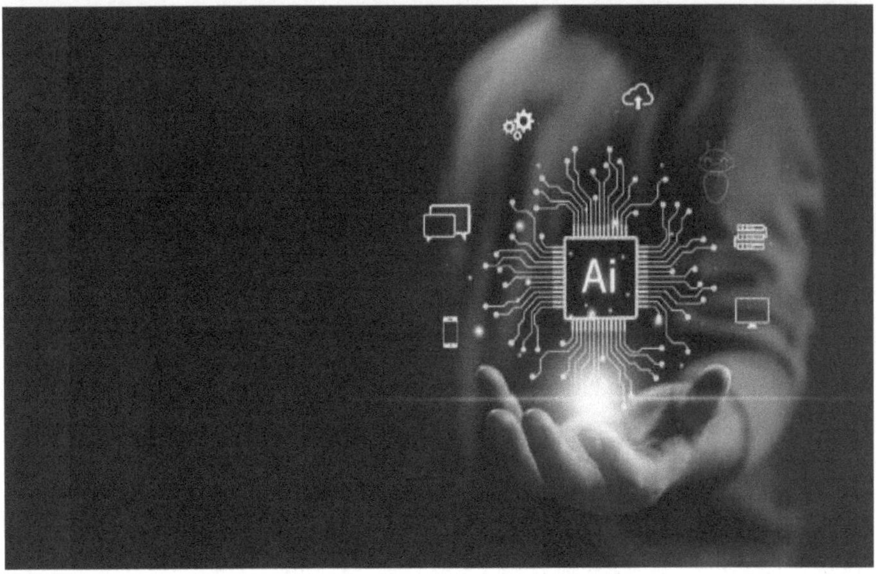

CHAPTER ONE

INTRODECTION

1.1 What is Artificial Intelligence?

Artificial Intelligence (AI) is the field of computer science dedicated to solving cognitive problems typically associated with human intelligence, such as learning, creativity, and image recognition. Modern organizations collect large amounts of data from various sources such as smart sensors, human-generated content, monitoring tools, and system logs. The goal of artificial intelligence is to create self-learning systems that extract meaning from data. AI can then apply that knowledge to solve new problems in human-like ways. For example, AI technology can respond meaningfully to human conversations, generate authentic images and text, and make decisions based on real-time data inputs. Your organization can integrate AI capabilities into your applications to improve your business processes, improve customer experiences, and accelerate innovation.

1.2 The Concept of Artificial Intelligence

The concept of Artificial Intelligence is related to the intelligence associated with digital or electronic devices such as; Computer, cellular devices or robots, and artificial intelligence expresses the ability of these digital devices to perform tasks associated with intelligent beings. The term artificial intelligence applies to systems that have human intellectual processes such as; The ability to think, discover meaning and learn from past experiences. Examples of operations performed by digital devices that are due to the presence of artificial intelligence include: Discovering proofs of mathematical theorems, playing chess, medical diagnosis, web search engines, voice or handwriting recognition.

In the past six months, Chatbots, like ChatGPT, and image creators, like midjourney, have become a cultural phenomenon.

But artificial intelligence or "machine learning" models have been around for quite some time.

1.3 What is the Difference Between Artificial Intelligence and Machine Learning?

Simply put, machine learning is a sub-part of the artificial intelligence system, and expresses the ability of a machine to think without being programmed externally. How is that?

Well, conventional machines are usually programmed with a number of rules about how to behave or operate within a given context, through a set of if-then-else instructions. But machine learning technology allows devices to continue to think and develop based on the data they receive in different circumstances and contexts.

1.4 How has Artificial Intelligence Technology Developed?

Artificial intelligence has gone through many stages from its beginnings to the present day, so it is important to have a general idea about the stages of development of artificial intelligence over the years. The following is a summary of the most important of these events:

The first time the word "robot" was mentioned dates back to 1921 when the Czech writer Karl Čapek used it in his play "Rossum's International Robots." The word is derived from "robota," which means work.

Likewise, the history of artificial intelligence goes back to the classical philosophers in Greece, and the study of the issue of the existence of artificial intelligence began in 1940 AD in a school of thought called Connectivism, where the process of thinking in it began to be studied, and Alan Turing presented a research paper in which he studied a thinking machine that imitates humans without any noticeable differences in it. In 1950 AD. Hodgkin Huxley came to present a research paper entitled "Computing Machines and Intelligence," a model that simulates the human brain in the form of an electrical network representing neurons, and an electrical current that simulates the impulses that turn on or off cells. These models and studies helped launch the concept of artificial intelligence in 1956 AD at a conference held by the College of Technology. Dartmouth. Between 1957 and 1974, advances in computing allowed computers to store more data and process it faster. During this period, scientists developed machine learning (ML) algorithms. Advances in this field led agencies such as the Defense Advanced Research Projects Agency (DARPA) to create an AI research fund. Initially, the main goal of this paper was to explore whether computers could transcribe and translate spoken language.

During the 1980s, development was facilitated by enhanced funding and an expansion of the set of algorithmic tools used by scientists in artificial intelligence. David Rumelhart and John Hopfield published research on deep learning techniques, which showed that computers can learn from experience.

From 1990 to early 2000, scientists achieved several basic AI goals, such as beating the world chess champion with the help of AI. With more computing data and more processing power in the modern era than in previous decades, AI research is now more common and more accessible. It is rapidly evolving into general artificial intelligence so that programs can perform complex tasks. Programs can create, make decisions, and learn on their own, tasks previously limited to humans.

The major achievement was in 2016 when Google developed an artificial intelligence program called AlphaGo, which was able to defeat the world champion in the complex board game Go. This achievement was a really big step in the field of machine learning because AlphaGo learned the rules of the game and was able to play at an expert level on its own without any previous programming.

The fields of artificial intelligence and its applications continued to develop in subsequent years as well, and its applications expanded into practical life. We saw the intelligent robot "Sophia" capable of building almost real relationships with humans, and artificial intelligence techniques were used in mobile phones through assistance applications such as Google Assistant or Siri and many others. Another aspect that we will discuss later in the article.

Today, we cannot say that there is a real existence of what is known as super artificial intelligence, or Super AI in English. But there is no doubt that this science is constantly evolving, and will witness further development and progress in the future.

1.5 How Artificial Intelligence Works

Artificial intelligence works in the digital environment through the availability of digital devices and specialized programs to analyze and design algorithms, and machine learning. In general, the artificial intelligence system accommodates large amounts of training data. Training data is used to form associations and patterns that are later used to build future predictions, such as automated response in smart robots, the process of identifying objects in images and describing them by reviewing millions of examples saved by the smart device.

1.6 Types of Artificial Intelligence

AI is one of the fastest growing areas of technological development. However, today, even the most complex AI models only make use of "narrow AI," which is the simplest of the three types of AI. The other two are still the stuff of science fiction and, at the moment, are not being used in any practical way. Thus, at the rate computer science has advanced in the past 50 years, it is difficult to say where the future of artificial intelligence will take us.

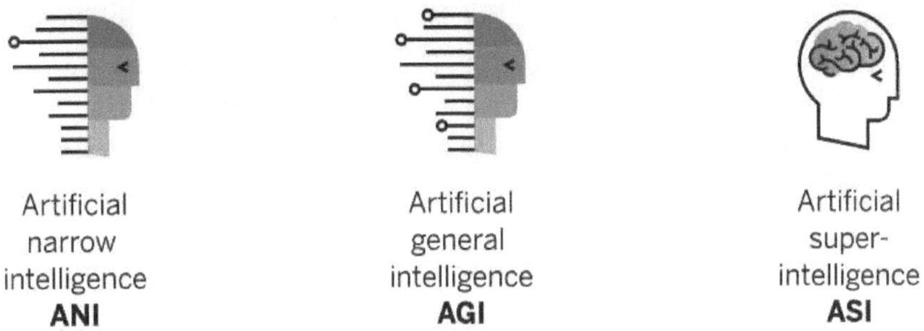

The Three Main Types of Artificial Intelligence

1.6.1 Artificial Narrow Intelligence (ANI)

ANI is the type of artificial intelligence that exists today and is also known as "weak" artificial intelligence. While the narrow tasks AI can perform may be driven by highly complex algorithms and neural networks, they are nonetheless singular and goal-oriented. Facial recognition, internet searches, and self-driving cars are all examples of the limitations of artificial intelligence. They are classified as weak not because they lack range and power, but because they are still far from possessing the human components that we attribute to true intelligence. Philosopher John Searle defines narrow AI as "useful for testing a hypothesis about minds, but which would not actually be minds."

Narrow artificial intelligence focuses on performing one type of task, but very well, so that it focuses on executing one task professionally. But it operates under far more constraints than human intelligence. An example of narrow artificial intelligence is the Google search engine. Image recognition software. Personal assistants, such as Alexa and Siri. Self-driving cars.

1.6.2 Artificial General Intelligence (AGI)

(Artificial General Intelligence) Artificial general intelligence is also known as strong artificial intelligence, and it is a type of intelligence found in smart machines and devices. Artificial general intelligence is characterized as a type of intelligence found in a machine that gives it general intelligence like a human, so that this intelligence is used to solve... No problem. Examples of devices that have general artificial intelligence include: Robots that are used to accomplish many tasks and make decisions based on the situation, but building robots that have human-like intelligence is still difficult and requires building large and complex neural networks like those found in the brain. Types of artificial intelligence The following are the types of artificial intelligence:

Reactive machines: Reactive machines are known as the simplest existing level of robot, as they are a machine designed to deal with one type of data and respond to current situations only. They are machines that are unable to create memories or use current information to build and make future decisions to improve their level or Developing its intelligence, it is only designed to respond to the current situation. Examples of interactive machines include; Machines designed to play chess against humans, such as Deep Blue from IBM, are designed to respond to the player's movements by evaluating the pieces on the chessboard and moving them according to their encoded playing strategies.

Limited memory: A limited memory machine is a machine capable of storing a limited number of information based on the data that the limited memory machine previously dealt with, so that the limited memory machine can build knowledge through memory when combined with its previously programmed data. Examples of machines that use limited memory include; Self-driving cars, as these cars store pre-programmed data such as; Maps or traffic signs, and comparing this stored data with information surrounding the car such as; Speed and directions of nearby vehicles and side-by-side pedestrian movement and take appropriate action based on this data.

Theory of Mind The theory of mind was used in designing the famous robot Sophia, a robot capable of using information to interact with situations in a human-like manner, which would teach the machine or robot how to act in a different and new situation. The theory of mind in the development and design of robots that are used as Chatbots is based on the human mind, which is based on the feelings and thoughts that a person has before he makes the decision-making process, so that the theory of mind robot Sophia talks to humans, and uses information and images in making decisions and responding to humans, in addition to... To show dazzling facial expressions.

Self-awareness Self-awareness devices are the ultimate goal of the existence of artificial intelligence, and they are devices that do not currently exist. These machines have human-level mental awareness and understand why they exist in this world, so that the machine does not just ask for something it needs, but understands that it needs Something, this means that the machine deeply understands its internal state and can predict the feelings of others around it just like humans. For example, when a person screams in front of us, we realize that he is angry, and this conclusion is based on the feelings that the person himself feels, so these conclusions go back to the presence of the mind.

An AGI must be able to successfully perform any intellectual task that a human can perform. Like narrow AI systems, AGI systems can learn from experience and can identify and predict patterns – but they have the potential to go a step further. AGI can extrapolate that knowledge across a wide range of tasks and situations that neither previously acquired data nor existing algorithms have addressed.

The top supercomputer is one of only a few such supercomputers in the world that denotes AGI. It can perform 200 quadrillion calculations in one second – which would take a human a billion years to do. For AGI models to be meaningful, they will not necessarily need that much power, but they will require computational capabilities that currently exist only at supercomputer levels.

1.6.3 Artificial Super Intelligence (ASI)

In theory, ASI systems are completely self-aware. Beyond simply simulating or understanding human behavior, they understand it on a fundamental level.

Empowered by these human traits—and augmented even more with processing and analysis power far beyond our own—ASI could seem to offer a scientific dystopian future in which humans become increasingly obsolete.

It is unlikely that anyone living today will see such a world, but it does mean that artificial intelligence is advancing at a rate that makes it important to consider ethical guidelines and oversight in anticipation of an artificial intelligence that could surpass us in almost every measurable way. As Stephen Hawking advises, “Because of the great potential of artificial intelligence, it is important to investigate how to reap its benefits while avoiding potential pitfalls.”

1.7 Historical Overview

The first concept of a "thinking" machine appeared in the writings of the ancient Greeks. Writers and filmmakers have used "machine intelligence" in science fiction and futurist novels and films.

Its features began to emerge in the modern era, when Alan Turing published a research paper in 1950 entitled "Computing Machinery and Intelligence", asking "Can machines think?" He then presented the "Turing Test", in which he tried to distinguish between computer responses and human text.

In 1956, John McCarthy coined the term "artificial intelligence" at the first ever artificial intelligence conference at Dartmouth College. In the same year, Allen Newell, J. C. Shaw, and Herbert Simon created the "Logic Theorist" program, the first artificial intelligence program.

In 1967, Frank Rosenblatt created the "Mark I Perceptron" machine, the first computer based on a neural network that "learns" through trial and error.

A year later, Marvin Minsky and Seymour Papert published a book called Perceptron, which became a landmark work on perceptrons, a type of artificial network developed in the early 1950s and 1960s.

In the 1980s, neural networks began using the backpropagation algorithm to “train” themselves, and were widely used in artificial intelligence applications, and are a key component of deep learning.

In 1995, Stuart Russell and Peter Norvig published Artificial Intelligence: A Modern Approach, which became one of the leading textbooks in the field.

IBM’s Deep Blue later defeated world champion Garry Kasparov in a chess match in 1997, and John McCarthy published a paper called What is Artificial Intelligence? in 2004, proposing a definition of it as “the science and engineering of making intelligent machines.”

In 2011, IBM's Waston computer beat champions Ken Jennings and Brad Rutter on Merv Griffin's CBS television game show Jeopardy!.

In 2015, Baidu's Minoa supercomputer used a special type of "deep neural network" called a "convolutional neural network" (known as artificial intelligence technology) that uses deep learning to identify and classify images with a higher accuracy rate than the average human.

In 2016, Google's DeepMind AI program AlphaGo beat South Korean professional Lee Sedol, a professional at the traditional Asian game of Go, in a five-game match.

This ancient game is famous for its complexity, as it relies on strategy and intuition and is open to many possibilities, and many in the field believed that no machine could excel at it.

AlphaGo was programmed with millions of moves from previous masters of the game, so it could predict its chances of winning and adjust its game plan accordingly. Then the DeepMind team launched another program called AlphaGo Zero, which did not give it any additional instructions, but it was able to teach itself by playing against itself. Within three days, AlphaGo Zero was able to defeat all copies of AlphaGo, and within 40 days it was able to independently discover the principles of the game that took humanity thousands of years to discover. The computer also developed new strategies of its own.

Then artificial intelligence began to enter people's public life, and was used in smart vacuum cleaners and cooking appliances, in modern self-driving cars, in smart watches and modern phones and what they contain of "voice assistants" such as "Siri" on iPhones and "Bixby" for Samsung users. The launch of the "Chat GPT" program in 2022 led to a huge change in the performance of artificial intelligence and its new generative capabilities, as it began to imitate humans and provide information based on a large database, and was able to perform professions and skills that were always specific to humans.

The limits of artificial intelligence did not stop at this point, but it began to generate images, videos, and audio texts read in different forms and voices according to the data requested from it, and it is now used to produce complete works that required months of work in a short time, threatening the disappearance of many professions.

1.8 Ambition and Warning

The ambition of scientists and researchers in the field of artificial intelligence does not stop at a limit, and reaches its peak when they talk about the possibility of manufacturing a mind with super intelligence that exceeds human ability, and they also talk about artificial consciousness or feeling.

In the midst of happiness with what has been achieved and looking forward to what will be achieved in this field, a team of scientists warns that this may mean the dominance of machines and the disappearance of the role of humans, and British astrophysicist Stephen Hawking said that complete artificial intelligence in the sense of creating computers that have their own minds "could herald the end of the human race." Tesla founder Elon Musk considers artificial intelligence “the greatest threat to our existence as humans,” and likens thinking machines to “nuclear weapons” and “the devil.”

Swedish philosopher Nick Bostrom, who works at Oxford University, conducted a poll among a group of artificial intelligence experts about the date when they believe that science will achieve a high level of machine intelligence. These scientists expressed their belief that this will be achieved on average in 2075, and after 30 years from that, machines with super-intelligent intelligence can be created that can outperform human thinking, and 21% of those included in the poll said that this will never happen. As for Yoshua Bengio, a professor of computer science at the University of Montreal in Canada, he believes that we should not worry about intelligent technologies, as they need many years of slow and gradual development before they reach the extent that can be feared, because their development is based on sciences and ideas that are still in their infancy. Ethical Challenges

Machines remain a human industry, which may be affected by people's religious, cultural and moral background, so many institutions and countries require developers in this field to take into account several principles to maintain a balance between the vast technological leaps and the basic rights of users, including:

Integrity and fairness, to prevent any bias or discrimination between individuals, groups and categories, and several smart chat programs have fallen into this when asked about political and religious issues that caused anger among their users, so program developers began teaching them to refuse to answer sensitive issues and respond with "I am still learning how to answer this question".

Privacy and security, through protecting the privacy of personal data, and cybersecurity standards, with the aim of preventing unauthorized access to data, which may lead to damage to reputation or psychological, financial or professional damage.

Humanity, as artificial intelligence systems are supposed to be built with a fair and ethical methodology based on human rights and basic cultural values. Systems must be designed so that they do not deceive, manipulate or create behavior that is not intended to empower and enhance human skills.

Social and environmental benefits, by enhancing the positive and beneficial impact of social and environmental priorities for the benefit of individuals and society as a whole, and not causing harm to individuals and societies.

Reliability and safety, by ensuring that the AI system adheres to the specified specifications, and works according to the mechanism intended by its designers, not for hidden purposes.

Transparency and interpretability, by building AI systems with a high degree of clarity and interpretability, with features to track the stages of automated decision-making, especially those that may lead to harmful effects on individuals.

Accountability and responsibility, so that designers, developers and AI system administrators bear moral responsibility for decisions and actions that may lead to potential risks and negative effects on individuals and societies.

Human oversight, governance and appropriate management must be applied throughout the entire life cycle of the AI system to ensure that there are appropriate mechanisms to avoid harm and prevent the misuse of this technology.

AI systems should not deceive people or unjustifiably harm their freedom of choice, and that designers, developers and people implementing the AI system should be mentioned and accessible to those who want to communicate with them.

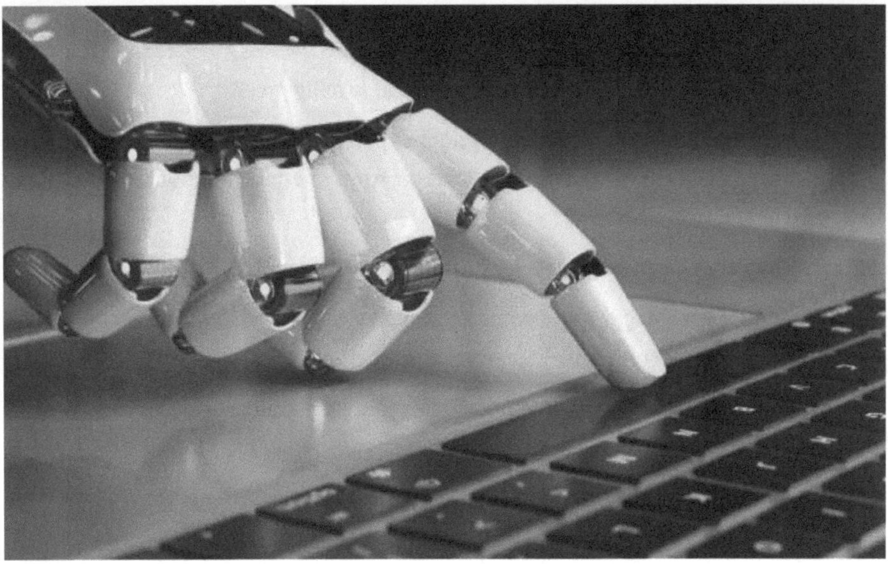

CHAPTER TWO

ADVANTAGES AND DISADVANTAGES OF ARTIFICIAL INTELLIGENCE

2.1 Advantages and Disadvantages of Artificial Intelligence

Everything has benefits, but they are often accompanied by drawbacks and harms. Below is an explanation of the advantages and disadvantages of artificial intelligence:

2.1.1 What are the disadvantages of artificial intelligence?

Its applications are expensive. Limited experts working in the field of artificial intelligence. Inability to transfer information from one task to another. It requires deep technical expertise.

2.1.2 What are the advantages of artificial intelligence?

Reducing time spent performing data-heavy tasks. Deliver consistent results. Introducing AI-powered virtual agents.

Artificial Intelligence has the potential to provide a range of benefits to various sectors.

1. Overcoming complex problems

AI technology can use machine learning and deep learning networks to solve complex problems with human-like intelligence. AI can process information at scale, by encountering patterns, identifying information, and providing answers. You can use AI to solve problems in a range of areas such as fraud detection, medical diagnostics, and business analytics.

2. Increase business efficiency

Unlike humans, AI technology can work 24/7 without degrading performance. In other words, AI can perform manual tasks flawlessly. You can let AI focus on repetitive and boring tasks, so you can use human resources in other areas of the business. Artificial Intelligence can reduce employees' workloads while facilitating all business-related tasks.

3. Make smarter decisions

AI can use machine learning to analyze large amounts of data faster than any human can. AI platforms can identify trends, analyze data, and provide guidance. By making predictions from the data, AI helps suggest the best course of action for the future.

4. Automation of business processes

You can train AI using machine learning so that it can perform tasks accurately and quickly. This can increase operational efficiency by automating parts of the work that employees struggle to do or find tedious. Likewise, you can use AI automation to free up employee resources to do more complex and creative work.

2.2.How Does Artificial Intelligence Learn?

The machine learning process is called training, where a computer program is provided with a large amount of data, sometimes with labels that explain what the data is and a set of commands.

Commands might be, for example: "Find all images that contain faces" or "Sort these sounds."

The program will then look for patterns in the data provided to it to respond to these commands.

The process of training artificial intelligence may need some modifications or additions, such as "This is not a face" or "These two voices are different," but what the program learns from the data and clues that are presented to it becomes a model for the artificial intelligence, and the training material is finished until its capabilities are determined.

One way to look at how the training process can create different types of artificial intelligence is to think about the evolution of different animals.

Over millions of years, the natural environment has contributed to animals developing specific abilities, and in a similar way, the millions of cycles that artificial intelligence takes while being fed its training data will shape the way it evolves and lead to specialized models of artificial intelligence.

2.3 What are the Practical Applications of Artificial Intelligence?

Artificial intelligence has a wide range of uses. While it's not an exhaustive list, here's a collection of examples that highlight various AI use cases.

a. Process documents intelligently

Intelligent Document Processing (IDP) translates unstructured document formats into usable data. For example, it converts business documents such as emails, images, and PDF files into structured information. Intelligent Document Processing (IDP) uses artificial intelligence techniques such as natural language processing (NLP), deep learning, and computer vision to extract, classify, and validate data.

For example, HM Land Registry processes title deeds for more than 87 percent of land in England and Wales. Case learners at HMLR compare and review complex legal documents relating to property transactions. The organization deployed an AI application to automate the document comparison process, reducing review time by 50 percent and increasing approval of ownership transfers.

b. Monitor application performance

Application performance monitoring (APM) is the process of using software tools and telemetry data to monitor the performance of business-critical applications. AI-based APM tools use historical data to predict problems before they occur. It can also solve problems in real-time by suggesting effective solutions to your developers. This strategy keeps applications running efficiently and addresses bottlenecks.

For example, Atlassian produces products aimed at facilitating teamwork and organization. Atlassian uses AI-based APM tools to continuously monitor applications, detect potential issues, and identify prioritized risks. With this functionality, teams can quickly respond to machine learning-powered recommendations and overcome performance drops.

c. Predictive maintenance

AI-enhanced predictive maintenance is the process of using large amounts of data to detect problems that may lead to the failure of processes, systems, or services. Predictive maintenance allows companies to address potential problems before they occur, reducing downtime and preventing disruptions.

For example, Baxter uses 70 manufacturing sites around the world and operates 24/7 to deliver medical technology. Baxter uses predictive maintenance to automatically detect abnormal conditions in industrial equipment. Users can implement effective solutions early to reduce downtime and improve operational efficiencies.

d. Medical research

Medical research uses artificial intelligence to streamline processes, automate repetitive tasks, and process vast amounts of data. You can use AI technology in medical research to streamline the end-to-end drug discovery and development process, transcribe medical records, and improve time to market for new products.

A real-world example is C2i Genomics using AI to power highly customizable genomic pathways and clinical tests. By covering computational solutions, researchers can focus on clinical performance and method development. Engineering teams are also using AI to reduce engineering resource and maintenance requirements and reduce non-recurring engineering (NRE) costs.

e. Business analytics

Business analytics uses artificial intelligence to collect, process, and analyze complex data sets. You can use AI analytics to predict future values, understand the root cause of data, and reduce time-consuming processes.

For example, Foxconn uses AI-enhanced business analytics to improve forecast accuracy. It achieved an 8 percent increase in forecast accuracy, resulting in annual savings of $533,000 at its plants. They also use business analytics to reduce wasted labor and increase customer satisfaction by making data-driven decisions.

2.4 What are the Main AI Technologies?

Deep learning neural networks form the core of artificial intelligence techniques. It mimics the processing that occurs in the human brain. The brain contains millions of neurons that work together to process and analyze information. Deep learning neural networks use artificial neurons that process information together. Each artificial neuron, or ganglion, uses mathematical calculations to process information and solve complex problems. This deep learning approach can solve problems or automate tasks that typically require human intelligence.

2.5 Types of Artificial Intelligence

Today, artificial intelligence is divided into four basic types, very similar to Maslow's hierarchy of basic needs. The simplest types of artificial intelligence can only perform basic functions, while the most advanced types are an entity that is fully aware of itself and what is going on around it, and is similar to... To a large extent human consciousness.

These four types are as follows:

1. Reactive Machines.
2. Limited Memory.
3. Theory of Mind.
4. Self-Awareness

Today, we have passed the stage of the first type of it, and we are on the verge of mastering and professionalizing the second type, but the third and fourth types of artificial intelligence exist only as a theory, and they will most likely represent the next stage of the development of artificial intelligence.

2.6 Let's Take A Closer Look at these Four Types and What Each one Means:

1. Reactive Machines

Interactive machines perform only basic tasks, and this type of artificial intelligence is the simplest of all. Machines that use this type respond to some inputs with some outputs, and their operating mechanism does not involve any self-learning process.

We can say that it is the first stage of artificial intelligence, examples of which include simple devices that recognize the face, for example. Or DeepBlue, a computer that was able to defeat the world chess champion.

2. Limited Memory

In this type, artificial intelligence has the ability to store data or previous expectations and use them to make better predictions in the future. With limited memory, engineering and building machine learning techniques becomes more complex.

Examples of machines that use this type of artificial intelligence are self-driving cars, which store various data related to the condition of the roads, other cars on the road, and other factors, and based on this data, they make decisions about the route they will take or the specific reaction they will take.

It is worth saying that most of the devices today that rely on artificial intelligence use limited memory, including personal assistance applications such as Google Assistance, voice and image recognition programs, chatbots, and others.

3. Theory of Mind

While there are many machines that use previous types of artificial intelligence, this type is still only a theoretical idea, or a project that is still being developed.

We can say that the theory of mind is the next stage of artificial intelligence systems that scientists are currently working on creating and developing. In this type, the machine (thanks to artificial intelligence technology) will be able to understand the entities it interacts with, know their needs, feelings, principles, and even the thinking process it undertakes.

In order to understand the difference between this type and the previous one, let us imagine that you are driving your car to an important meeting, but the traffic jam was stifling, which made you lose your nerve.

You might angrily yell at Google Maps for a shortcut, but the app won't offer you any moral support, such as saying, "This is the quickest way we can go. Do you want me to call someone to apologize or postpone the meeting for a while?"

Google Maps will continue to show the same results based on its road reports and data.

However, by using theory of mind technology, this application will be a better companion for you, it will understand your feelings and thoughts and help you feel better, which is what is now being developed and worked on within the field of artificial emotional intelligence or Artificial Emotional Intelligence.

4. Self Awareness

Finally, in a distant, unknown future, humans may finally be able to develop self-aware artificial intelligence. It is the same entity that we see in science fiction films. This type of artificial intelligence may raise many hopes, but it also raises many fears. The idea of a self-aware robot with a special, independent intelligence is troubling, because that means that humans would then have to negotiate with the machine they created with their own hands, and the outcome of these negotiations opens room for many assumptions, expectations, and fantasies.

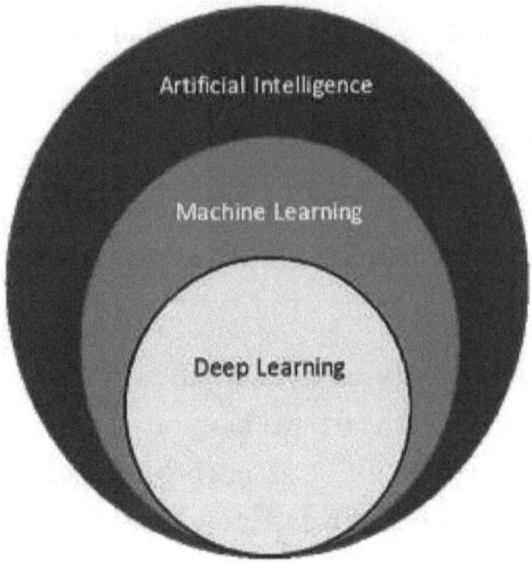

You can develop different AI techniques by training deep learning neural networks in different ways. Below we discuss some of the main techniques based on neural networks:

a. Natural language processing

Natural Language Processing (NLP) uses deep learning algorithms to interpret, understand, and gather meaning from textual data. Natural language processing (NLP) can process human-generated text, which makes it useful for summarizing documents, automating chatbots, and performing sentiment analysis.

b. Computer vision

Computer vision uses deep learning techniques to extract information and insights from videos and images. Using computer vision, a computer can understand images just as a human can understand them. You can use computer vision to monitor online content for inappropriate images, recognize faces, and classify image details. In self-driving cars and trucks, it is very important to monitor the environment and make split-second decisions.

2.7 Benefits and Challenges of AI Implementation

There are many success stories that demonstrate the value of AI. Companies that add machine learning and cognitive interaction to traditional business processes and applications can dramatically improve user experience and boost productivity.

However, there are some obstacles. Few companies have deployed AI at scale, for a number of reasons. For example, unless they use cloud computing, machine learning projects are often very expensive. They are also complex to build and require expertise that is in high demand and in short supply. Knowing when and where to integrate these projects, as well as when to outsource, will help mitigate these challenges.

2.8 AI Success Stories

AI is the driver behind some notable success stories. According to the Harvard Business Review, the Associated Press produced 12 times more stories by training an AI program to write short stories about earnings. The effort freed up the agency's journalists to write more in-depth articles.

Deep Patient, an AI tool developed by the Icahn School of Medicine at Mount Sinai, allows doctors to identify high-risk patients before they are diagnosed with diseases. The tool analyzes a patient's medical history to predict nearly 80 diseases up to a year before they appear, according to insideBIGDATA.

2.9 Off-the-shelf AI Makes it Easier to Implement AI

The emergence of AI-powered solutions and tools means more companies can leverage AI at a lower cost and in less time. Off-the-shelf AI refers to solutions, tools, and programs that either have AI capabilities built in or automate algorithmic decision-making.

Off-the-shelf AI includes self-healing databases and pre-built models for recognizing images and analyzing text in different datasets.

2.10 How to Get Started with AI

Connecting with Customers with Chatbots Chatbots use natural language processing to understand customers and allow them to ask questions and get information. They can also learn over time so they can add more value to customer interactions.

Data center monitoring. IT operations can simplify monitoring with a cloud-based platform that integrates all data and automatically tracks boundaries and anomalies.

Conduct business analysis without the need for experts. Analytical tools with a visual user interface allow non-technical people to easily navigate through the system and get understandable answers.

2.11 Creating the Right Culture

Making the most of AI, and avoiding the pitfalls that prevent successful implementations, means creating a culture across teams that fully supports the AI ecosystem. In this type of environment

Business analysts work with data scientists to define problems and goals

Data engineers manage the data and the data platform, so that it is fully operational for analytics

Data scientists prepare, explore, visualize, and model data on a data science platform

IT engineers manage the underlying infrastructure needed to support data science at scale, whether on-premises or in the cloud

Application developers deploy models into applications to create data-driven products

Discover how data science teams can work together more efficiently

2.12 From AI to Adaptive Intelligence

As AI capabilities reach core enterprise operations, a new term has emerged: adaptive intelligence. Adaptive intelligence applications help companies make better business decisions by combining the power of real-time internal and external data with decision science and high-level computing infrastructure.

Essentially, these applications make your business smarter. This in turn enables you to provide your customers with better products, recommendations, and services, all of which lead to better business outcomes.

Learn more about the transformative power of Oracle SaaS applications with embedded AI

2.13 AI as a strategic imperative and competitive advantage

AI is a strategic imperative that drives greater efficiency, new revenue opportunities, and increased customer loyalty. It is rapidly becoming a competitive advantage for many organizations. With AI, companies can accomplish more in less time, create personalized and engaging customer experiences, and predict business outcomes to increase profitability.

But AI is still a new and complex technology. To get the most out of it, you need expertise in how to build and manage AI solutions at scale. An AI project requires more than just hiring a data scientist. Companies must implement the tools, processes, and management strategies to ensure AI success.

2.14 Best Practices for Getting the Most Out of AI

Harvard Business Review offered the following recommendations for getting started with AI:

Apply AI capabilities to activities that have the greatest and immediate impact on revenue and cost.

Use AI to boost productivity with the same number of people, rather than adding or eliminating staff.

Start implementing AI in the back office, not the front office (you'll benefit greatly from applying it to IT and accounting).

2.15 Get help with your AI experience

There's no opting out of the AI transformation. To stay competitive, every company must eventually embrace AI and create an AI ecosystem. Companies that fail to embrace AI in some capacity over the next 10 years are bound to fall behind.

While your company may be the exception to this rule, most companies don't have the skills and in-house expertise to develop the kind of ecosystem and solutions that can leverage AI capabilities.

For a successful AI transformation journey that includes strategy development and access to tools, look for a partner with domain expertise and a comprehensive AI portfolio.

2.16 AI Learning Library

What is data science?

Companies are actively combining statistics with computer science concepts like machine learning and artificial intelligence to extract insights from big data to drive innovation and transform decision-making.

What is machine learning?

Machine learning, a subset of artificial intelligence (AI), focuses on creating systems that learn from data to automate and speed up decision-making and reduce the time to value.

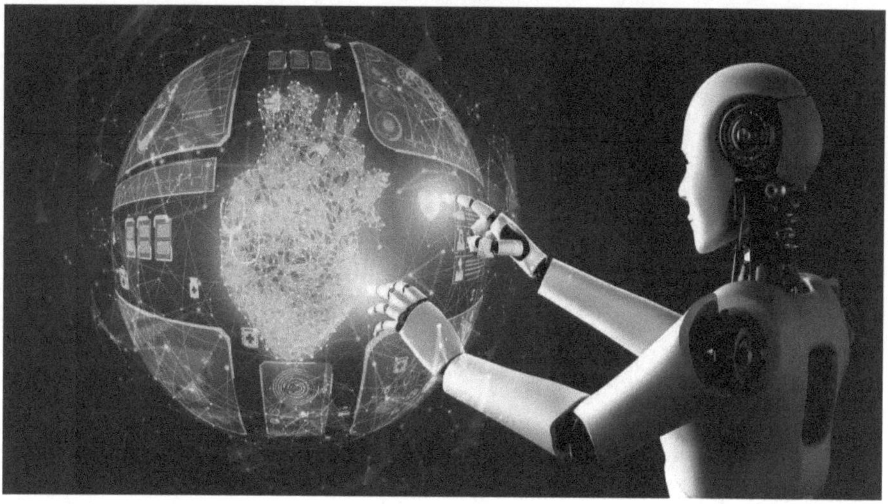

CHAPTER THREE

GENERATIVE ARTIFICIAL INTELLIGENCE

3.1 Generative Artificial Intelligence

Generative AI refers to artificial intelligence systems that can create new content and new elements such as images, videos, text, and audio from simple text commands. Unlike previous AI that was limited to data analysis, generative AI leverages deep learning and massive data sets to produce high-quality, innovative creative output that resembles what a human would produce. While enabling exciting creative applications, there are concerns about bias, harmful content, and intellectual property. Overall, generative AI represents a major advance in AI's capabilities to create new content and new elements in a way similar to what humans create.

3.2 What are the Main Components in an AI Application Architecture?

The architecture of artificial intelligence consists of four basic layers. Each of these layers uses different technologies to fulfill a specific role. Below is an explanation of what happens at each layer.

First layer: data layer

Artificial intelligence relies on various techniques such as machine learning, natural language processing, and image recognition. Data is at the center of these technologies, and forms the foundational layer of AI. This layer mainly focuses on preparing data for AI applications. Modern algorithms, especially those based on deep learning, require huge computational resources. Therefore, this layer includes hardware that acts as a sublayer, providing the basic infrastructure for training AI models. You can access this layer as a fully managed service from a third-party cloud provider.

Second layer: machine learning frameworks and algorithm layer

Engineers and data scientists create machine learning frameworks to meet the requirements of specific business use cases. Developers can then use pre-built functions and classes to easily build and train models. Examples of these frameworks include TensorFlow, PyTorch, and scikit-learn. These frameworks are vital components of the application architecture and provide essential functionality to easily create and train AI models.

The third layer: the model layer

In the model layer, the application developer implements the AI model and trains it using data and algorithms from the previous layer. This layer is pivotal to the decision-making capabilities of the AI system.

Here are some of the main components in this layer.

a. Model structure

This architecture defines the capability of the model, as it includes layers, neurons, and activation functions. Depending on the problem and resources, one can choose from feed-forward neural networks, convolutional neural networks (CNNs), or other networks.

b. Model parameters and functions

Values acquired during training, such as neural network weights and biases, are essential for predictions. The Loss Function evaluates the performance of the model and aims to minimize the discrepancy between the predicted output and the real output.

c. Optimization tool

This component adjusts the model parameters to minimize the loss function. Different optimization tools such as gradient descent and adaptive gradient algorithm (AdaGrad) serve different purposes.

Fourth layer: application layer

The fourth layer is the application layer, which is the customer-facing part of the AI architecture. You can ask AI systems to complete certain tasks, generate information, provide information, or make data-driven decisions. The application layer allows end users to interact with AI systems.

3.3 What are the Challenges Facing Implementing AI?

AI faces a number of challenges that make implementation more difficult. The following obstacles are examples of the most common challenges facing implementing and using AI.

1. Data Governance

Data governance policies must adhere to regulatory restrictions and privacy laws. To implement AI, you must manage data quality, privacy, and security. You are responsible for customer data and privacy protection. To manage data security, your organization must have a clear understanding of how AI models use and interact with customer data across every layer.

2. Technical difficulties

Training AI using machine learning consumes enormous resources. For deep learning techniques to function, a high level of processing power is necessary. You must have a robust computing infrastructure to run AI applications and train your models. Processing power can be expensive or limit the scalability of your AI systems.

3. Data limitations

To train unbiased AI systems, you need to input huge amounts of data. You must have enough storage capacity to handle and process the training data. Likewise, you must be proficient in governance and data quality processes to ensure the data you use in training is accurate.

3.4 Uses and Fields of Artificial Intelligence

The applications and fields of artificial intelligence are expanding to include many aspects of our lives, and there is no doubt that each of us has dealt with artificial intelligence technologies in one way or another during our daily lives.

Artificial intelligence applications

Artificial intelligence is used in many important technological and life applications, which has facilitated many aspects of life and performed various functions that were limited to the human mind alone. Among the most important applications of artificial intelligence are the following:

1. Robotics, which is used in many industries such as healthcare, finance, and marketing.

2. Customer service, such as robots that are used to respond to customer chats, and robots that perform customer service and electronic marketing functions.

3. Digital media that displays ads that are of interest to the target person by analyzing his data and understanding his trends from his searches on the Internet.

4. Facial recognition This technology is used in many devices such as a smartphone, and it works to learn and perceive patterns to produce quick and effective results.

5. Virtual voice assistants help and imitate human intelligence through voice communication.

6. Fitness applications Examples of fitness applications that use artificial intelligence include smart watches that count steps, calculate calories, and other applications concerned with fitness.

7. Artificial intelligence in marketing

Marketing is an effective way to beautify products in order to attract more customers. We humans are really good at beautifying our products and marketing them, but what if there was an algorithm (computer program) or robot that was created for the purpose of marketing only?! He will do a great job without a doubt.

Let's think together: several years ago, finding a product on an e-commerce site without knowing its exact name was a real nightmare and an almost impossible task.

But today, as soon as we search for a specific product, e-commerce sites will show us all other similar goods. It has become as if search engines are reading our thoughts, and within a few seconds you can find information and products that would have taken days and weeks to find in the past.

One of the important practical applications of using artificial intelligence in marketing is what we see on the famous Netflix website.

Do you know why many people love this site? And they find it very easy to find a suitable movie for them?

The reason is that Netflix uses highly accurate predictive technology, based on the viewer's behavior and reaction to the films he watches or chooses, and then suggests programs that are compatible with your previous choices.

8. Artificial intelligence in banking services

Artificial intelligence in banking is growing exponentially beyond expectations, with many banks already adopting AI-based systems to provide customer support and detect anomalies and credit card fraud. Like HDFC Bank in India.

HDFC Bank has developed an AI-based chatbot called EVA (Electronic Virtual Assistant), and since its launch Eva has handled more than 3 million customer queries, interacted with more than half a million and conducted more than a million conversations. Eva can collect information from thousands of sources and provide simple answers in less than half a second!

Artificial intelligence technologies are also used to prevent fraud by tracking the use of bank cards and analyzing the behavior of bank transactions to identify fraud and fraud attempts, which is what major companies such as MasterCard do.

9. Artificial intelligence in healthcare

Many organizations and medical care centers rely on artificial intelligence to treat patients and save the lives of millions. There are many examples of this:

Cambio Health Care has developed a clinical support system for stroke prevention that sends warning alerts when a patient is at risk of having a cardiac arrest.

Coala Life has also developed a smart digital device that can detect heart diseases.

Aifloo is developing a system to track the performance of people in nursing homes and home care and help them carry out their activities and routines.

Perhaps the best thing about using artificial intelligence technologies in the field of health care is that there is no need to develop any new medicines, but rather all that is needed is to use existing medicines in a correct and intelligent way that saves lives.

10. Artificial intelligence in the field of space exploration

Space missions and discoveries constantly require the analysis of huge amounts of data. Artificial intelligence and machine learning are the best ways to handle and process data at this scale.

Astronomers have been able to use artificial intelligence techniques to study and analyze data collected by the Kepler telescope over the years. Thanks to this, they have been able to identify and discover galaxy systems, solar systems, and planets that are thousands and millions of light years away from us.

Artificial intelligence applications are also used in probes and spacecraft that roam the planet Mars and discover its secrets.

This is not all, as all recent discoveries in this field are the result of the use of modern artificial intelligence techniques.

11. Artificial intelligence in education

Although it is still too early to see human-like robots assuming the role of teacher and giving lectures and lessons, there are undoubtedly many uses of artificial intelligence in the field of education that help students and teachers alike achieve the greatest possible benefit from the learning process. Examples:

Personalized Learning: Where artificial intelligence techniques are used to customize the educational experience for individuals by analyzing their learning styles, previous experiences, and abilities, and then determining the appropriate educational materials for them.

Assisting teachers in performing some administrative tasks such as conducting assessments, preparing tests, or managing related logistical matters.

Breaking down geographical barriers by making global classrooms accessible to everyone, regardless of their language, location, or any other obstacles, as artificial intelligence technologies contribute to overcoming these barriers.

12. Speech recognition

Speech recognition software uses deep learning models to interpret human speech, identify words, and discover meaning. Neural networks can convert speech into text and indicate vocal emotions. You can use speech recognition in technologies such as virtual assistants and call center software to identify meaning and perform related tasks.

Speech recognition is an interdisciplinary subfield of computer science and computational linguistics that develops methodologies and technologies that enable the recognition and translation of spoken language into text by computers. It is also known as automatic speech recognition (ASR), computer speech recognition or speech-to-text (STT). It incorporates knowledge and research in the computer science, linguistics and computer engineering fields. The reverse process is speech synthesis.

Some speech recognition systems require "training" (also called "enrollment") where an individual speaker reads text or isolated vocabulary into the system. The system analyzes the person's specific voice and uses it to fine-tune the recognition of that person's speech, resulting in increased accuracy. Systems that do not use training are called "speaker-independent" systems. Systems that use training are called "speaker dependent".

Speech recognition applications include voice user interfaces such as voice dialing (e.g. "call home"), call routing (e.g. "I would like to make a collect call"), domotic appliance control, search key words (e.g. find a podcast where particular words were spoken), simple data entry (e.g., entering a credit card number), preparation of structured documents (e.g. a radiology report), determining speaker characteristics, speech-to-text processing (e.g., word processors or emails), and aircraft (usually termed direct voice input). Automatic pronunciation assessment is used in education such as for spoken language learning.

The term voice recognition or speaker identification refers to identifying the speaker, rather than what they are saying. Recognizing the speaker can simplify the task of translating speech in systems that have been trained on a specific person's voice or it can be used to authenticate or verify the identity of a speaker as part of a security process.

From the technology perspective, speech recognition has a long history with several waves of major innovations. Most recently, the field has benefited from advances in deep learning and big data. The advances are evidenced not only by the surge of academic papers published in the field, but more importantly by the worldwide industry adoption of a variety of deep learning methods in designing and deploying speech recognition systems.

There are many uses, some of which are:

There are many uses and applications of artificial intelligence, including:
In-car systems

Education

Health care: Medical documentation

Therapeutic use

Military: High-performance fighter aircraft

Helicopters

Training air traffic controllers

Telephony and other domains

People with disabilities

Aerospace (e.g. space exploration, spacecraft, etc.) NASA's Mars Polar Lander used speech recognition technology from Sensory, Inc. in the Mars Microphone on the Lander.

Automatic subtitling with speech recognition

Automatic emotion recognition

Automatic shot listing in audiovisual production

Automatic translation

eDiscovery (Legal discovery)

Hands-free computing: Speech recognition computer user interface

Home automation

Interactive voice response

Mobile telephony, including mobile email

Multimodal interaction

Real Time Captioning

Robotics

Security, including usage with other biometric scanners for multi-factor authentication

Speech to text (transcription of speech into text, real time video captioning, Court reporting)

Telematics (e.g. vehicle Navigation Systems)

Transcription (digital speech-to-text)

Video games, with Tom Clancy's EndWar and Lifeline as working examples

Virtual assistant (e.g. Apple's Siri)

Accuracy of speech recognition may vary with the following:

Vocabulary size and confusability

Speaker dependence versus independence

Isolated, discontinuous or continuous speech

Task and language constraints

Read versus spontaneous speech

Adverse conditions

3.5 Models, Methods, and Algorithms

Both acoustic modeling and language modeling are important parts of modern statistically based speech recognition algorithms. Hidden Markov Models (HMMs) are widely used in many systems. Language modeling is also used in many other natural language processing applications such as document classification or statistical machine translation.

1. **Hidden Markov Models**

Modern general-purpose speech recognition systems rely on hidden Markov models. These are statistical models that produce a sequence of symbols or quantities. Hidden Markov models are used in speech recognition because the speech signal can be considered as a discrete, stationary signal or a short-term, stationary signal. On a short time scale (e.g., 10 ms), speech can be approximated as a stationary process. Speech can be considered a Markov model for many purposes.

Another reason for the popularity of hidden Markov models is that they can be trained automatically, and are simple and computationally feasible to use. In speech recognition, a hidden Markov model outputs a series of n-dimensional real-valued vectors (where n is a small integer, such as 10), and outputs one of these vectors every 10 milliseconds. The vectors consist of cepstral coefficients, which are obtained by taking the Fourier transform of a short time window of speech and uncorrelating the spectrum using a cosine transform, then taking the first (most significant) coefficients. A hidden Markov model tends to have in each case a statistical distribution that is a mixture of diagonal variance Gaussians, which will give a probability for each observed vector. Each word, or (for more general speech recognition systems) each phoneme, will have a different output distribution; a hidden Markov model for a series of words or phonemes is created by concatenating the individual trained hidden Markov models for the separate words and phonemes.

One possible improvement to decoding is to keep a set of good candidates rather than just the best candidate, and to use a better scoring function (rescoring) to evaluate these good candidates so that we can choose the best according to this revised score. The set of candidates can be kept either as a list (the N-best list approach) or as a subset of models (a network). Rescoring is typically done by trying to minimize Bayesian risk (or an approximation of it). Instead of taking the source sentence with maximum likelihood, we try to take the sentence that minimizes the expectation of a given loss function with respect to all possible versions (i.e. we take the sentence that minimizes the average distance to the other possible sentences weighted by its estimated probability). The loss function is typically the Levinstein distance, although it can be different distances for specific tasks; the set of possible versions is of course pruned to maintain processability. Efficient algorithms have been devised to rescore networks represented as weighted finite state transformers with edit distances that themselves represent a finite state transformer to check certain assumptions..

2. Dynamic time warping (DTW)-based speech recognition

Dynamic time warping is a technique that was historically used for speech recognition but has now been largely superseded by a more successful HMM-based approach.

Dynamic time warping is an algorithm for measuring the similarity between two sequences that may differ in time or speed. For example, similarities in walking patterns can be detected, even if a person in one video is walking slowly and another is walking faster, or even if there is acceleration and deceleration during the course of a single observation. DTW has been applied to video, audio, and graphics - in fact, any data that can be converted to a linear representation can be analyzed using DTW.

Automatic speech recognition was a well-known application, dealing with different speaking speeds. In general, it is a method that allows a computer to find a perfect match between two given sequences (for example, a time series) with certain constraints. That is, the sequences are "warped" non-linearly to match each other. This sequence alignment method is often used in the context of hidden Markov models.

3. Neural networks

Neural networks emerged as an attractive approach to acoustic modeling in speech recognition in the late 1980s. Since then, neural networks have been used in many aspects of speech recognition such as phoneme classification, phoneme classification through multi-objective evolutionary algorithms,isolated word recognition, audiovisual speech recognition, audiovisual speaker recognition, and speaker adaptation.

Neural networks make fewer explicit assumptions about the properties of feature statistics than HMMs and have several qualities that make them more attractive recognition models for speech recognition. When used to estimate the probabilities of a part of speech features, neural networks allow for discriminative training in a natural and efficient manner. However, despite their effectiveness in classifying short-term units such as individual phonemes and isolated words, early neural networks were rarely successful in continuous recognition tasks due to their limited ability to model temporal dependencies.

One approach to deal with this limitation has been to use neural networks as a preprocessing step, feature transformation or dimensionality reduction, prior to homogeneous matrix model-based recognition. However, recently, LSTM and related recurrent neural networks (RNNs), time-delay neural networks (TDNN's), and transformers have shown improved performance in this area.

4. Deep feedforward and recurrent neural networks

Deep neural networks and denoising autoencodersare also under investigation. A feed-forward deep neural network (DNN) is an artificial neural network with multiple hidden layers of units between the input and output layers. Similar to shallow neural networks, deep neural networks can model complex nonlinear relationships. Deep neural network architectures generate compositional models, where additional layers enable features to be built up from lower layers, giving tremendous learning capacity and thus the potential to model complex patterns of speech data.

The success of deep neural networks in large-vocabulary speech recognition occurred in 2010 by industrial researchers, in collaboration with academic researchers, where large output layers of the deep neural network were based on context-dependent HMMs generated by decision trees. See comprehensive reviews of this development and the state of the art as of October 2014 in the recent Springer book from Microsoft Research. See also the background related to automatic speech recognition and the impact of different machine learning models, including deep learning in particular, in recent overview articles.

One of the fundamental principles of deep learning is to eliminate hand-crafted feature engineering and use raw features. This principle was first successfully explored in a deep autoencoder architecture on "raw" spectrogram or linear filter bank features, showing its superiority over Mel-Cepstral features that have a few stages of fixed transformation from spectrograms. It has recently been shown that true "raw" speech features, waveforms, produce excellent results for speech recognition at a larger scale.

5. End-to-end automatic speech recognition

Since 2014, there has been significant research interest in "end-to-end" automatic speech recognition. Traditional acoustics-based approaches (i.e. all HMM-based models) require separate components and training for the speech, voice, and language model. Holistic models jointly learn all components of the speech recognition software. This is valuable because it simplifies the training and deployment process. For example, an n-gram language model is required for all HMM-based systems, and a typical n-gram language model often takes up several gigabytes of memory, making it impractical to deploy on mobile devices. Consequently, modern commercial automatic speech recognition systems from

Google and Apple (as of 2017) are deployed in the cloud and require a network connection rather than on-device local. The first attempt at end-to-end automatic speech recognition using systems based on connectional temporal classification (CTC) was presented by Alex Greaves of Google DeepMind and Navdeep Jaitley of the University of Toronto in 2014. The model consists of recurrent neural networks and a CTC layer. The RNN-CTC model jointly learns pronunciation and the acoustic model together, however it is unable to learn language due to conditional independence assumptions similar to HMM. Thus, CTC models can directly learn how to map speech phonemes to English letters, but the models make many common spelling errors and must rely on a separate language model to clean up the texts. Baidu later expanded the work to very large datasets and demonstrated some commercial success in Mandarin Chinese and English. In 2016, the University of Oxford introduced LipNet, the first sentence-level lip-reading model from start to finish, using spatiotemporal convolutions coupled with an RNN-CTC architecture, surpassing human-level performance on a constrained grammar dataset. A large-scale CNN-RNN-CTC architecture was introduced in 2018 by Google DeepMind achieving six times better performance than human experts.

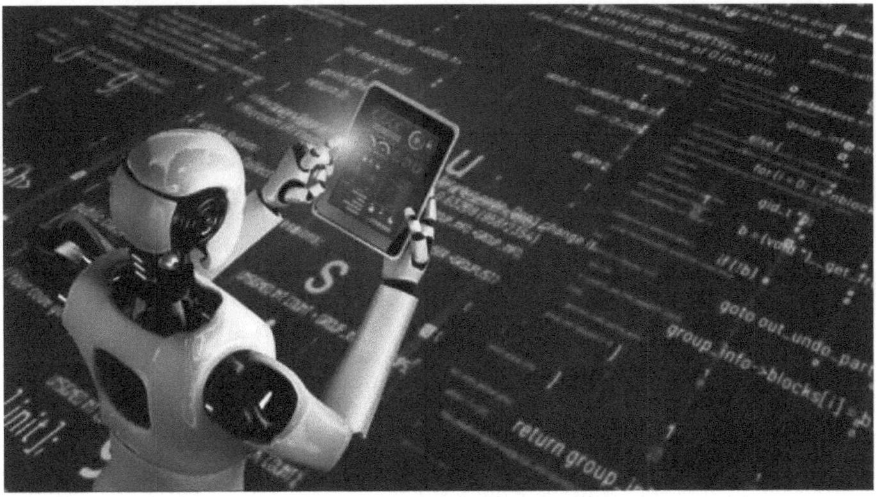

CAPTER FOUR

THE FUTURE OF ARTIFICIAL INTELLIGENCE AND ITS FUNCTIONS

4.1 The Future of Artificial Intelligence and its Functions

According to a study, artificial intelligence technology is expected to create 12 million additional jobs compared to the jobs it is expected to replace.

Thus, the concept of artificial intelligence has become more widespread and its fields and applications have expanded greatly in recent years. Which may lead us to ask: What is the future of artificial intelligence? What are its functions?

Answering these two questions will require two other more extensive and detailed articles from us, which you will already find on our website, where you can get to know better the concept of artificial intelligence as a university major, its most important axes, and its current and future prospects through the detailed description of the artificial intelligence major through the majors guide.

4.2 What are Chatbots?

Imagine the chatbot is a type of parrot. He imitates and can repeat words he has heard with a limited understanding of their context but without a full sense of their meaning.

Chatbots are doing the same, albeit on a more complex level, and are about to change our relationship with the written word.

But how do chatbots know how to write?

They are types of artificial intelligence known as large language models (LLMs) and are trained by feeding them massive amounts of text.

Large language models (LLM) are able to look at words and in full sentences and compare the use of words and phrases in one passage to other examples across all of their training data.

Using billions of comparisons between words and phrases, AI can read and answer a question, like typing text messages on your phone that predicts the word you want to type but on a large scale.

The amazing thing about large language models is that they can learn the rules of a language and discover the meaning of words without human help.

Expert point of view: The future of Chatbots

"In 10 years, I think we'll have chatbots that act like an expert in whatever field you want. So you'll be able to ask an expert doctor or an expert teacher or an expert lawyer, and whatever you need comes through having these systems do things for you."

Sam Altman - CEO of Open AI, creators of ChatGPT

Can I talk to artificial intelligence?

If you've used Alexa, Siri, or any other type of voice recognition system, you're using artificial intelligence.

Imagine a rabbit with large ears, adapted to pick up subtle differences in sound.

AI records sounds as you speak, removes background noise, separates your speech into phonemes, the individual sounds that make up a spoken word, and then matches them to a library of language sounds.

Your speech is then converted into text where any errors can be corrected during listening before providing you with the answer.

This type of artificial intelligence is known as natural language processing.

It's the technology behind everything from saying "yes" to confirm a phone banking transaction, to asking your mobile phone to tell you the weather for the next few days in the city you're traveling to.

Can artificial intelligence understand images?

Has your phone ever collected your photos into folders with names like “At the Beach” or “At Night Out”?

So you've been using AI without realizing it. The AI algorithm has unveiled the nature of your photos and collected them for you.

These programs are trained by recognizing a large set of images, all labeled with a simple description.

If you submit images to be processed by AI to recognize, for example, images with the name “bike,” the AI will begin to determine what a bike looks like and how it differs from a boat or a car.

Sometimes, AI is trained to detect small differences within similar images.

This is how facial recognition works, finding an exact relationship between the features on your face that make it special and unique when compared to any other face on the planet.

The same type of algorithms have been trained on medical scans to identify life-threatening tumors, and can work through thousands of scans in the time it might take a consultant oncologist to decide on just one.

How does artificial intelligence create new images?

Image recognition has recently been adapted into artificial intelligence models just as chameleons adapt their colors to their surroundings.

Innovative image AI systems can transform complex visual patterns gathered from millions of photos and graphics into entirely new images.

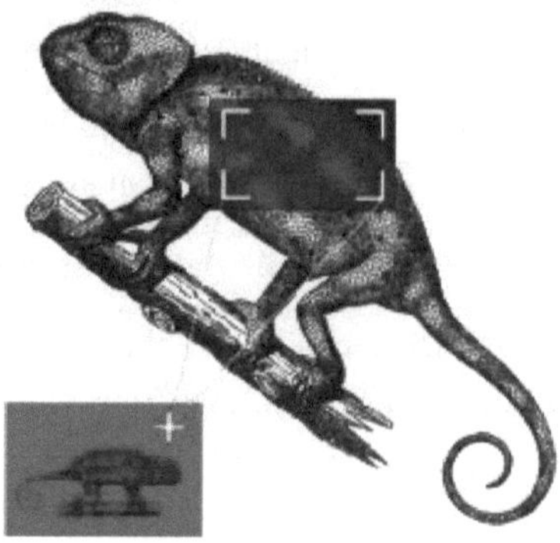

You can ask the AI to create a photograph of something that has never happened, for example, a photo of a person walking on Mars.

Or you can creatively direct the portrait: "Draw a portrait of an England football coach, drawn in the style of Picasso."

State-of-the-art AI systems begin the process of creating this new image with a set of pixels of random colors.

The AI looks at random points for any hint of a pattern it learned during training, such as building patterns for different objects.

These patterns are slowly improved by adding further layers of random points, keeping the points that develop the pattern and eliminating the useless ones, until finally similarity emerges.

For example, you develop and add all the necessary patterns and parts such as "Mars surface", "Astronaut" and "Walk", put them together and then you will get a new image.

Because the new image is built from layers of random pixels, the result is something that didn't exist before but is still based on billions of patterns the AI learned from the original training images.

The community is now beginning to discuss the impact of AI on copyright and business ethics in the production of artwork based on the hard work of real artists, designers, and photographers.

What about self-driving cars?

Self-driving cars have been part of the discussion around artificial intelligence for decades, cemented by science fiction in the popular imagination.

Artificial intelligence related to self-driving cars is done by equipping cars with cameras, radar, and lasers to sense the range.

Think of a dragonfly, which has a 360-degree angle of view and sensors on its wings to help it maneuver and make constant adjustments in flight.

In a similar way, an AI model uses data from its sensors to identify objects and know if they are moving, and if so, what type of object is moving, such as another car, a bike, a pedestrian, or something else.

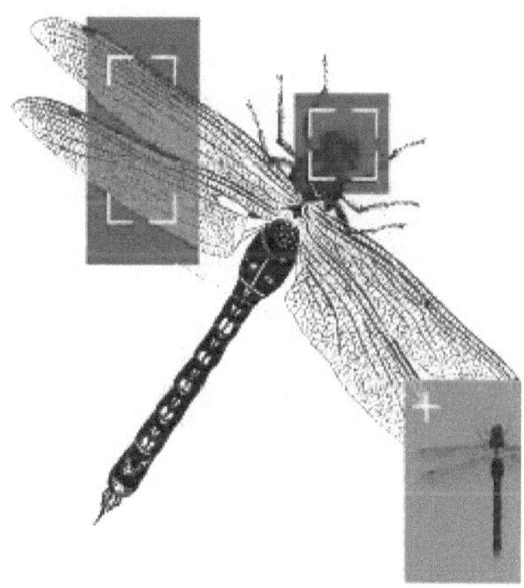

Thousands of hours of training have enabled AI to understand what good driving looks like by making real-world decisions and actions to drive a car and avoid collisions and accidents.

Predictive algorithms may have struggled for years to deal with the unpredictable nature of human drivers, but self-driving cars have now collected millions of data by being trained on real roads. In San Francisco, self-driving vehicles have started transporting passengers.

Autonomous driving is also a very general example of how new technologies can overcome even technical obstacles.

Government legislation and safety regulations, along with a deep sense of concern about what happens when we hand control over to machines, all remain potential barriers and obstacles to an automated future.

Expert opinion: Safer than humans

“I think where we want to get to is we want safer roads. It's an interesting thing that we're talking about now, especially when humans and robots are relatively close in performance. But over the next couple of years, given the rate of improvement that these systems have seen, I think this debate will become a thing of the past because they will be so much better than humans and we won't even have this debate.”

Kyle Vogt - CEO of Cruise Autonomous Vehicles

What does artificial intelligence know about you?

Some artificial intelligence systems deal with numbers and combine them to create huge amounts of information, and what emerges from this information is of great value.

There are likely already many profiles of your financial and social transactions, especially those you carry out online, that can be used to make predictions about your behavior

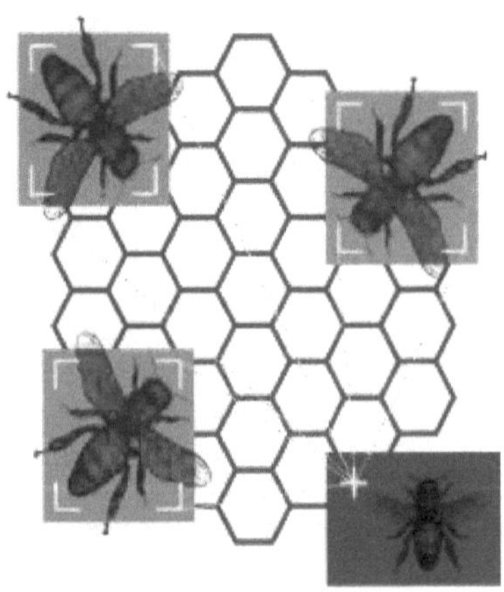

Your Shopping Card tracks your habits and tastes through your weekly purchasing pattern. Credit agencies keep track of how much you have in the bank and what you owe on your credit cards.

Netflix and Amazon track how many hours of content you watched last night. Your social media accounts will know how many videos you commented on today.

You are not alone, these numbers and data are available to everyone, which enables artificial intelligence models to use them to search for social trends.

AI models are already shaping your life, from helping decide whether you can get a loan or mortgage, to influencing what you buy by choosing which ads you see online.

Will artificial intelligence be able to do everything?

Is it possible to combine some of these skills into a single AI model?

This is exactly what one of the latest developments in artificial intelligence does.

It is called multimodal AI and it allows the model to look at different types of data such as images, text, audio or video and discover new patterns between them.

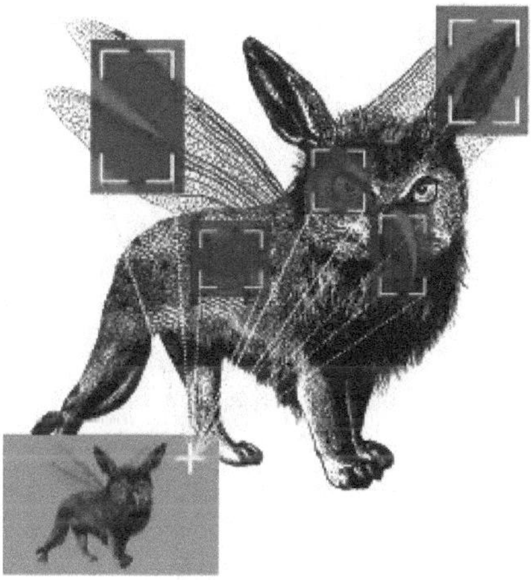

This multi-modal approach was one of the reasons for the huge jump in ability that ChatGPT demonstrated when its AI model was updated from GPT3.5, which was only trained on text, to GPT4, which was also trained on images.

The idea of a single model of artificial intelligence capable of processing any type of data and thus performing any task, from translating between languages to designing new drugs, is known as artificial general intelligence (AGI).

For some, this is the ultimate goal of all AI research. For others, it's a path to all those real-life science fiction events in which we unleash an intelligence so far beyond our understanding that we can no longer control it.

How do you train artificial intelligence?

Until recently, the key process in training most AI systems was known as "supervised learning."

Huge sets of training data were given labels by humans and AI was asked to detect patterns in the data.

The AI was then asked to apply these patterns to some new data and provide feedback on their accuracy.

For example, imagine giving the AI dozens of images – six labeled "car" and six labeled "pickup."

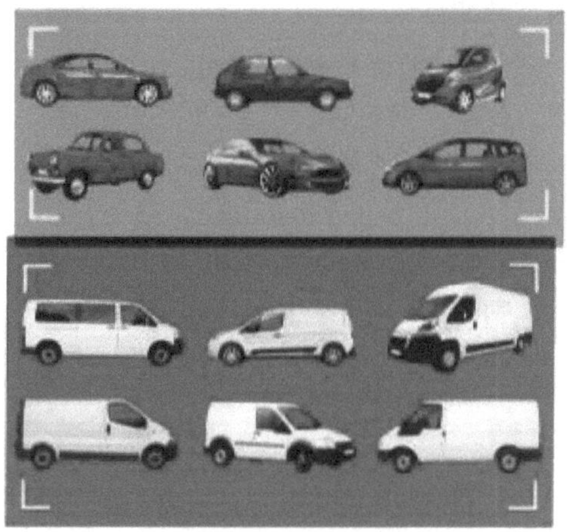

Next, have the AI create a visual pattern that sorts cars and vans into two groups.

Now, what do you think will happen when you ask him to classify this photo?

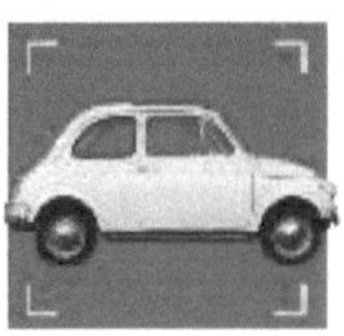

Unfortunately, the AI seems to think this is a pickup truck, which is not very smart.

Now show him this

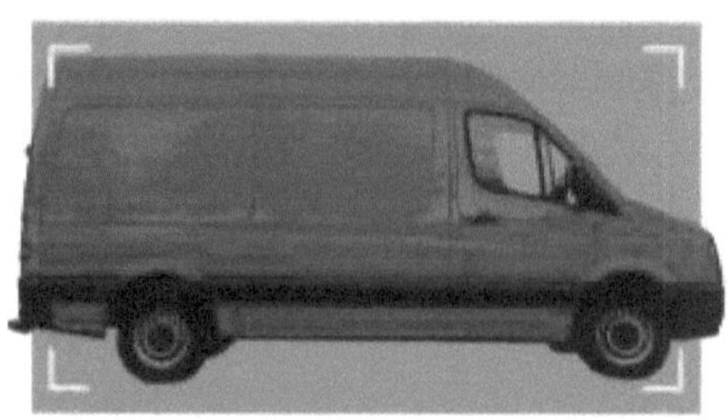

He will tell you that this is a car.

It's quite clear what went wrong.

From the limited number of images it was trained on, the AI determined that color was the strongest way to separate cars from pickup trucks.

But the amazing thing about the AI program is that it made this decision on its own – and we can help it improve its decision-making process.

We can tell him that he incorrectly identified the two new objects, and this will force him to find a new pattern in the pictures.

But more importantly, we can correct the bias in our training data by giving it more diverse images.

These two simple actions taken together, and at scale, are how most AI systems are trained to make incredibly complex decisions.

How does artificial intelligence learn on its own?

Supervised learning is effectively a powerful training method, but many recent advances in artificial intelligence are made possible by unsupervised learning.

In simpler terms, it is the use of complex algorithms and massive data sets that AI can learn without any human guidance.

ChatGPT is the most famous example.

The number of texts on the Internet and in digital books is so large that, over the course of several months, ChatGPT was able to learn how to combine words in a way that is meaningful in and of itself, with human intervention to adjust their responses.

Imagine that you have a large collection of books in a foreign language, some of which may contain pictures.

Eventually you might realize that the same word appeared on the page whenever there was a drawing or picture of a tree, and another word when there was a picture of a house.

You will notice that there was often a word similar in meaning to another of those words.

ChatGPT did this kind of careful analysis of the relationship between words to build a huge statistical model that it could then use to create new sentences.

It relies on huge amounts of computerized information that allows artificial intelligence to memorize a huge number of words, whether they are separate words, in groups, in sentences, or across pages. The artificial intelligence then reads and compares how the words are used over and over again in a small fraction of a second.

The rapid advances made by deep learning models in the past year have prompted a new wave of enthusiasm and concern about the potential of artificial intelligence, and there is no sign of it slowing down.

The promises and warnings of science fiction seem to have suddenly crept up on us and we find that we are already living in a world where artificial intelligence is beginning to reveal its strange, non-human abilities.

Expert opinion: Treat artificial intelligence on the principle of raising children

The answer to how we prepare machines for this morally complex world lies in the way we raise our children and prepare them to face our complex world. When we raise children, we don't know exactly the situations they will face. We do not provide them with an answer to every question they ask us. Instead, we teach them how to find the answer themselves."

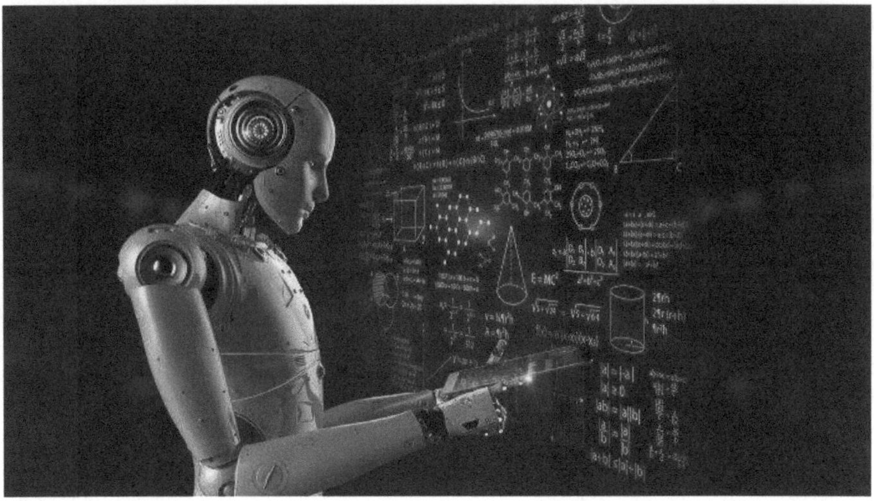

CHAPTER FIVE

ARTIFICIAL INTELLIGENCE TO SERVE HUMANITY AND THE WORLD

5.1 Artificial Intelligence to Serve Humanity and the World

Throughout history, man has searched for an invention that could mimic the human mind in its way of thinking. Artists, writers, filmmakers, and game developers alike have tried to find a logical explanation for the concept of artificial intelligence. For example, in 1872, Samuel Butler spoke in his novel "Erihon"

(1872) about machines and the great role they will play in developing humanity and moving the world to development and prosperity.

Over time, artificial intelligence has been present only in science fiction. Sometimes it highlights the potential benefits of artificial intelligence for humanity and its bright human aspects, and at other times it highlights the negative aspects expected from it, and it is portrayed as a fierce enemy of humanity who intends to usurp civilization and control. On her.

In 2018, artificial intelligence became a reality, not a fantasy, and no longer occupies a place only in the world of popular culture. The year 2018 was a major shift for artificial intelligence. This technology has grown significantly on the ground until it has become a major tool at the heart of all sectors.

Artificial intelligence has emerged from research laboratories and from the pages of science fiction novels, to become an integral part of our daily lives, from helping us navigate cities and avoid traffic jams, all the way to using virtual assistants to help us perform various tasks, and today our use of artificial intelligence has become rooted in... For the common good of society.

5.2 Using Artificial Intelligence for Good

Brad Smith, President and Chief Legal Officer at Microsoft, highlighted that the world was and is still suffering from ongoing humanitarian crises resulting from natural and human-caused disasters, and while these relief organizations seek to deal with these disasters and events, their work is still often nothing more than It is reactive, and difficult to scale.

According to Smith, artificial intelligence and data science, in addition to the expertise represented in environmental science and humanitarian aid, will help save more lives and alleviate suffering by improving methods that predict the occurrence and enhancing means of dealing with disasters before or after they occur.

Therefore, Microsoft launched the "AI for Earth" program, which aims to protect our planet through the use of data science. The duration of the program is five years and its cost is 50 million dollars, as the program disseminates Microsoft's experience, which reaches 35 years in the field of research. And technology in AI techniques in the four main sectors: agriculture, water, biodiversity and climate change.

"We believe that artificial intelligence can be a game changer in confronting pressing societal challenges and creating a better future," says Lucas Guba, who heads the AI for Earth program at Microsoft. "The African continent is considered the best place from which to see the radical changes of artificial intelligence, as it can... "Early adoption of artificial intelligence tools in areas such as agriculture and resource conservation will lead to environmental and economic benefits, from enabling the ability to better manage natural resources to upgrading the workforce."

5.3 The AI for Earth Program Aims to Protect the Planet Through Data Science

Industrialization is one of the most serious environmental problems facing our world today. For example, the climate changes that the world is witnessing, the pollution of soil and rivers, the large consumption of forest resources, and other environmental dangers are among the effects in which industrialization plays a fundamental role.

Fortunately, we have reached a unique and unprecedented point in human history. We are facing a new era known as the Fourth Industrial Revolution. This revolution has created a great opportunity for us to reshape the way we manage our environment today, as the capabilities of digitalization and societal transformations are harnessed in order to solve environmental problems. And creating a revolution in the field of sustainability.

Recognizing this unique opportunity, Microsoft and National Geographic announced a new partnership to advance research on major environmental challenges by harnessing the power of artificial intelligence. The AI for Earth Innovation Grant program has helped The newly launched $1.2 million grant will provide grants to 11 changemakers ranging from $45,000 to $200,000, with the aim of supporting their innovative projects in the areas of agriculture, water, biodiversity and climate change.

5.4 Artificial Intelligence Technologies

For AI to be useful, it must be workable. Its true value can only be realized when it provides actionable insights. If we think of AI in terms of the human brain, AI technologies are like hands, eyes, and body movements – everything that allows the brain's ideas to be implemented. Below are some of the most widely used and rapidly advancing artificial intelligence technologies.

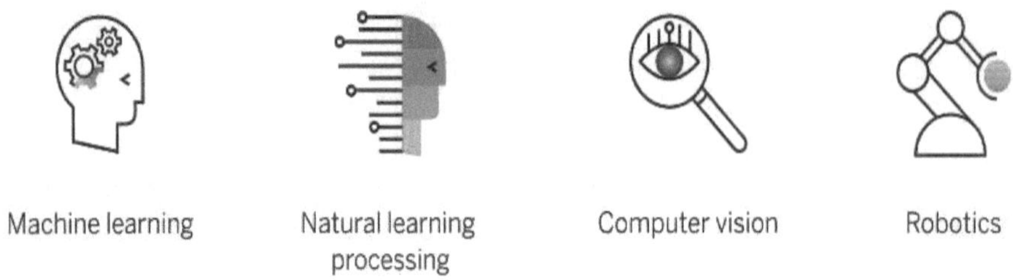

Artificial intelligence technologies

1. Machine training

Machine training – and all of its components – is a subset of artificial intelligence. In machine learning, algorithms are applied to different types of learning methods and analysis techniques, which allow the system to automatically learn and improve from experience without being explicitly programmed. For businesses, machine training can be applied to any problem or goal that requires predictive results, derived from complex data analysis.

What is the difference between artificial intelligence and machine training? Machine training is a component of AI and cannot exist without it. So it's not so much the case that they're different – as how they're different. Artificial intelligence processes data to make decisions and predictions. Machine learning algorithms allow AI to not only process that data, but use it to learn and get smarter, without the need for any additional programming.

2. Natural Language Processing (NLP)

NLP allows machines to recognize and understand written language, voice commands, or both. This includes the ability to translate human language into a form that an algorithm can understand. Natural Language Generation (NLG) is a subset of NLP that allows a machine to convert digital language into natural human language. In more sophisticated applications, NLP can use context to infer situation, mood, and other subjective qualities to more accurately interpret meaning. Practical applications of NLP include chatbots and digital voice assistants such as Siri and Alexa.

3. Computer vision

Computer vision is the way computers understand and "see" digital images and videos – as opposed to simply recognizing or classifying them. Computer vision applications use sensors and learning algorithms to extract complex, contextual information that can then be used to automate or inform other processes. Computer vision can also extrapolate data for predictive purposes which essentially means it can see through walls and around corners. Self-driving cars are a good example of computer vision in use.

4. Cybernetics

Robotics is not new and has been used for years, especially in manufacturing. But without applying AI, automation must be done through manual programming and calibration. If weaknesses or inefficiencies exist in those workflows, they can only be spotted after the fact – or after something breaks down. A human operator can often never know what has led to a problem, or what adaptations can be made to achieve better efficiency and productivity. When AI is brought into the mix – usually via IoT sensors – it brings with it the ability to dramatically expand the scope, size, and type of robotic tasks being performed. Examples of robots in industry include order picking robots for use in large warehouses and agricultural robots that can be programmed to pick or serve crops at optimal times.

5.5 Artificial Intelligence Ethics and Challenges

In 1948, computer science pioneer Alan Turing said: "A computer would deserve to be called intelligent if it could fool a human into believing that it is a human." Although the processing speed and analytical power of a modern AI-driven computer would have seemed unbelievable to Turing, he was nevertheless likely to understand the moral implications that this level of power offered. As artificial intelligence improves in our understanding and judgment, it appears increasingly human. As we generate increasing amounts of personal data through digital channels, we need more and more to be able to trust the AI applications that support so many of our daily activities. Here are some examples of ethical challenges that business leaders need to be aware of and monitor.

• Ethical use of customer data In the 2020s, the bulk of the information we share and collect as businesses or individuals is done through digitally connected channels. At the start of 2020, there were more than 3.5 billion smartphones in the world, all of which shared vast amounts of data – from their GPS location to the personal details and preferences of their users, via social media and search behaviours. As companies gain broader access to their customers' personal information, it becomes increasingly important to establish ever-evolving standards and protocols to protect privacy and minimize risks.

• AI Bias Bias can creep into an AI system due to human bias in programming its algorithms or through systemic biases that can be propagated via faulty assumptions in the machine learning process. At the first stage, it is clear to see how this could happen. But in the second, it can be difficult to identify and avoid. A well-known example of AI bias occurred within the US healthcare system, where AI applications were being used to personalize standards of care. The algorithm learned that certain demographic groups were less able to pay for care. Then extrapolate this information to mistakenly associate that group with being less fortunate in care. After discovering this unfortunate error, computer scientists at the University of California Berkeley worked with developers to adjust the algorithm variables, thus reducing bias by 84%.

• Transparency in AI and Explainable AI Transparency in AI is the ability to determine how and why an algorithm reached a particular conclusion or decision. The AI and machine training algorithms that inform the results – and the results themselves – are often too complex to be understood by humans. Algorithms like these are known as "black box" models. For companies, it is important to ensure that data models are fair, unbiased, and can be interpreted and externally audited. Especially in fields such as aviation or medicine, human lives are at stake. It is therefore vital that the humans who use this data take data governance initiatives very seriously.

• Deep Thoughts and Fake News Deepfault is a cross between "deep learning" and "fake." It is a technique that uses artificial intelligence and machine training to - typically - superimpose one person's face onto another person's body in a video, with such accuracy that it is indistinguishable from the original. In its innocent form, it can produce stunning visual effects such as removing 30 years from the lifespan of Robert De Niro and Joe Pesci in The Irishman. Unfortunately, its most common use is to create believable fake news stories or to put celebrities in charts or bargain videos in which they did not originally appear.

5.6 How Google Developed Artificial Intelligence

Committed to creating tools that benefit everyone, we developed a set of AI principles in 2018, which outline our goal of developing advanced technology that can responsibly address some of society's biggest challenges.

For example, we use AI to do the following:

• Support efforts to reduce climate change, such as reducing frequent traffic stops to reduce vehicle emissions

• Predict or monitor natural disasters, such as predicting floods in more than 20 countries and tracking the spread of wildfires in real time

• Supporting innovations in health care, such as facilitating tuberculosis screening and helping in early detection of breast cancer

Our Principles also outline areas in which we will not seek to use AI, such as technologies that cause public harm or violate international law and human rights.

5.7 Artificial Intelligence.. When the Machine Thinks

Artificial intelligence is a term given to the capabilities displayed by machines and programs, which simulate the mental capabilities of humans, such as learning, inference, and reaction to situations that were not programmed into the machine. It is also the name of an academic field concerned with how to create computers and programs capable of adopting intelligent behavior.

It is a prominent feature of the modern era, developed by humans to serve them in accomplishing their tasks with great accuracy, high speed, and solid reliability.

This achievement was accompanied by economic challenges that caused a huge gap in the distribution of wealth between developed and developing countries, and between individuals themselves in the same country, and it became a major threat to a number of jobs.

5.8 The Origin of the Name

The term artificial intelligence was introduced by the American computer scientist John McCarthy (1927-2011), who coined it in 1956, the year that witnessed the holding of a scientific conference at Dartmouth College in the United States to refer to the research being conducted at that time on the possibility of designing an intelligent machine capable of imitating and simulating human work.

At that conference, campaigns were announced to collect financial donations to support research in order to reach an invention similar to the human mind that enables machines to work on their own without the need for humans.

5.9 Great Leaps

Artificial intelligence is defined as the logical construction of software, algorithms and neural networks, which enables computerized machines to simulate human intelligence in learning, making decisions, solving problems, predicting outcomes, making recommendations and comparing options to achieve specific goals.

The development of programming languages and computer science has been an incentive to move forward in enhancing artificial intelligence to the point that it has become a science in its own right, combining many other sciences such as programming, logic, mathematics and even psychology and philosophy.

The development of artificial intelligence technology has achieved great leaps, and "deep learning" technology is its most prominent manifestation, which is based on developing artificial neural networks that mimic the way the human brain works, meaning that they are capable of experimenting, learning and developing themselves on their own without human intervention.

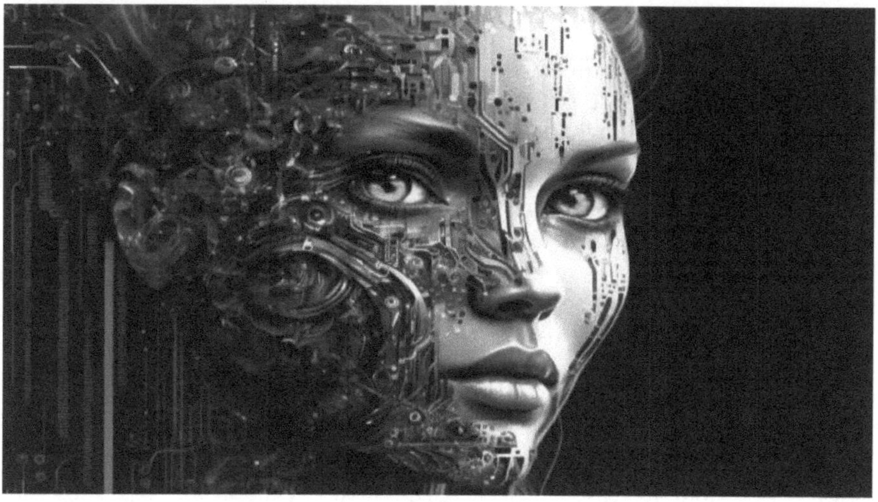

CHAPTER SIX

GENERATIVE ARTIFICIAL INTELLIGENCE

6.1 What is Generative Artificial Intelligence?

Generative AI is a type of artificial intelligence that can create new content and innovative ideas, including conversations, stories, photos, videos, and music. AI technologies attempt to mimic human intelligence in non-traditional computing tasks, such as image recognition, natural language processing (NLP), and translation. Generative AI represents the next step in artificial intelligence. You can train it to learn human language, programming languages, art, chemistry, biology or any complex subject. It reuses training data to solve new problems. For example, he can learn English vocabulary and create a poem from the words he processes. Your organization can use generative AI for various purposes, such as chatbots, media creation, product development and design.

6.2 Why is Generative AI important?

Generative AI applications, such as ChatGPT, have captured widespread attention and wild fantasies. This technology can help reinvent most customer and application experiences, create new applications never seen before, and help customers reach new levels of productivity.

According to Goldman Sachs, generative AI could lead to a 7 percent (or nearly $7 trillion) increase in global GDP. It also expects this technology to increase productivity growth by 1.5 percentage points over 10 years.

Below, we Present More Benefits of Generative AI.

1. Accelerate research

Generative AI algorithms can explore and analyze complex data in new ways. Therefore, researchers can discover new trends and patterns that may not be obvious otherwise. These algorithms can summarize content, identify multiple solution paths, brainstorm ideas, and create detailed documentation from research notes. This is why generative AI dramatically enhances research and innovation.

For example, generative AI systems are used in the pharmaceutical industry to create and optimize protein sequences and dramatically accelerate drug discovery.

2. Enhance customer experience

Generative AI can respond naturally to human conversation and act as a customer service tool and personalize customer workflows.

For example, you can use AI chatbots, voice bots, and virtual assistants to more accurately respond to customers in order to provide a solution from the first contact. They can increase customer engagement by presenting carefully selected offers and communicating in a personalized manner.

3. Improving business processes

With generative AI, your company can improve business processes leveraging machine learning (ML) and artificial intelligence (AI) applications across all lines of business. You can apply this technique across all lines of business, including engineering, marketing, customer service, finance, and sales.

6.3 For Example, here's what Generative AI can do to Improve:

a. Extracting data from any source and summarizing it for the purposes of cognitive research tasks

b. Evaluate different scenarios to reduce and improve costs in areas such as marketing, advertising, finance and logistics

c. Create synthetic data to create labeled data for supervised learning and other machine learning processes

d. Enhancing employee productivity

e. Generative AI models can grow employee workflows and serve as effective assistants for everyone in your organization. It can do everything from research to creativity in a human-like way.

6.4 Generative AI can Boost Productivity for Different Types of Workers:

a. Support creative tasks by creating multiple prototypes based on given inputs and constraints. It can also improve existing designs based on human feedback and specified constraints.

b. Create new code suggestions within application development tasks.

c. Support management by creating reports, summaries and forecasts.

d. Create new sales scripts, email content, and blogs for marketing teams

e. You can save time, reduce costs, and improve efficiency throughout your organization.

6.5 How will Generative AI Impact Industries?

Although generative AI can impact all industries over time, some industries are poised to quickly benefit from this technology.

1. Financial services

a. Financial services companies can harness the powers of generative AI to better serve their customers while reducing costs:

b. Financial institutions can use chatbots to create product recommendations and respond to customer inquiries, improving overall customer service

c. Lending institutions can speed up loan approvals for cash-strapped markets, especially in developing countries

d. Banks can quickly detect fraud attempts on claims, credit cards, and loans

e. Investment firms can harness the powers of generative AI to provide personalized financial advice to their clients at a low cost

2. Healthcare and life sciences

a. One of the most promising use cases for generative AI is accelerating drug discovery and research. Generative AI uses models to create new protein sequences with specific properties to design antibodies, enzymes, vaccines, and gene therapies.

b. Healthcare and life sciences companies can use generative models to design synthetic gene sequences for applications in synthetic biology and metabolic engineering. For example, they can create new biosynthetic pathways or improve gene expression for biomanufacturing purposes.

c. Finally, generative AI can be used to create synthetic patient and healthcare data. This is useful for training AI models, simulating clinical trials, or studying rare diseases without access to large real-world datasets.

3. Automotive and manufacturing

a. Automotive companies can use generative AI for many purposes, from engineering to in-vehicle experiences and customer service. For example, they can improve the design of mechanical parts to reduce drag in vehicle designs or adapt the design of personal assistants.

b. Automotive companies are using generative AI to provide better customer service by providing quick responses to the most common customer questions. Designs incorporating new materials, chips and parts can be created using generative AI to improve manufacturing processes and reduce costs.

c. Generative AI can also be used to generate synthetic data for testing applications. This is especially useful for data that is not often included in test data sets (such as defects or crashes in extreme use cases).

4. Media and entertainment

From animation and scripts to full-length films, generative AI models can produce new content at a fraction of the cost and time of traditional production.

6.6 Here are other ways you can use Generative AI in Industry:

a. Artists can supplement and enhance their albums with AI-generated tracks to create entirely new experiences

b. Media organizations can use generative AI to improve their audience experiences by delivering personalized content and personalized ads to increase revenue

c. Gaming companies can use generative AI to create new games and allow players to create avatars

6.7 Telecommunications

The first use cases for generative AI in the telecom sector focus on reinventing the customer experience. Customer experience is determined by subscribers' cumulative interactions across all touchpoints in the customer journey.

For example, telecommunications organizations can apply generative AI to improve customer service through human-like live chat agents. It can also improve network performance by analyzing network data to recommend fixes. It can reinvent customer relationships through personalized one-to-one sales assistants.

6.8 Energy

Generative AI is suitable for energy sector tasks that involve complex raw data analysis, pattern recognition, forecasting, and optimization. Energy organizations can improve customer service by analyzing enterprise data to identify usage patterns. Using this information, it can develop targeted product offerings, energy efficiency programs, or demand response initiatives.

Generative AI can help manage grids, increase site operational safety, and improve energy production through inventory simulation.

6.9 How does Generative AI Work?

As with all forms of AI, generative AI works using machine learning models, but these are very large models and pre-trained on huge amounts of data.

Incorporation forms

Foundation models (FM) are machine learning models trained on a wide set of generalized, unlabeled data. It is capable of performing a variety of general tasks.

Foundation models (FMs) are the result of the latest advances in technology that we have seen over the decades. In general, a foundation model uses learned patterns and relationships to predict the next element in a given sequence.

For example, when generating images, the model analyzes the image and creates a sharper, more accurate version of it. Likewise, with texts, the model predicts the next word in a text string based on the previous words and their context. It then chooses the next word using probability distribution techniques.

Big language models

Large Language Models (LLM) are one of the categories of Foundation Models (FM). For example, OpenAI's Generative Pre-Trained Transformer (GPT) models are large language models. Large language models focus in particular on language-based tasks, such as summarization, text generation, categorization, open-ended conversation, and information extraction.

What makes large language models special is their ability to perform multiple tasks. It can do this because it has many parameters that make it capable of learning advanced concepts.

A large language model, such as GPT-3, can consider billions of parameters and has the ability to generate content from very few inputs. As large language models are exposed before training to Internet-scale data in all its many different forms and myriad patterns, they learn to apply their knowledge in a wide range of contexts.

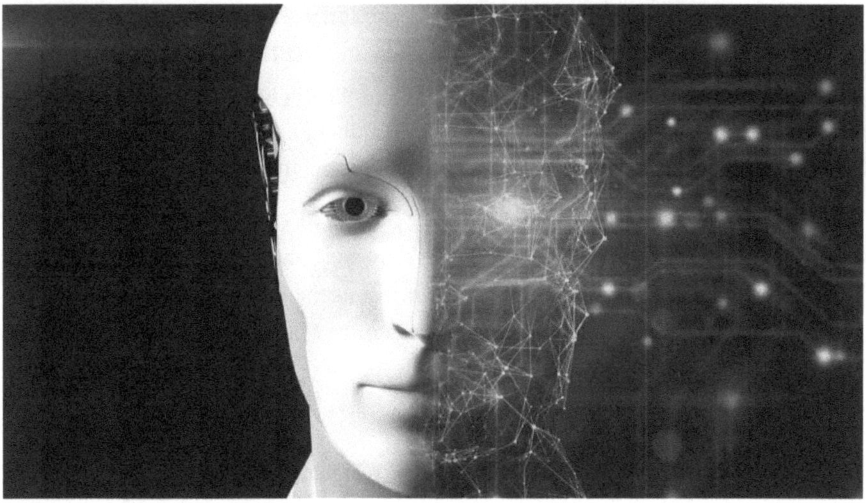

CHAPTE SEVEN

GENERATIVE AI MODELS

7.1 How do Generative AI Models Work?

Traditional machine learning models were discriminative or focused on classifying data points. She was trying to determine the relationship between known and unknown factors. For example, models look at images (the known data such as pixel arrangement, font, color, and shape) and map them to words (the unknown factor). Mathematically, models worked by specifying equations that could numerically map unknown and known factors such as the variables x and y.

The generative models perform another additional step. Instead of predicting a classification or label based on some given feature, it attempts to predict features based on some given classification or label. Mathematically, generative models calculate the probability of x and y occurring together. You learn the distribution of different data features and the relationships between them.

For example, generative models analyze images of animals to record variables such as different ear shapes, eye shapes, tail features, and skin patterns. You learn the features and relationships between them to understand what different animals generally look like. It can then recreate images of new animals that were not in the training set.

7.2 We Introduce Some Broad Categories of Generative AI Models.

a. Diffusion Models

Diffusion models create new data by repeatedly making controlled, random changes to an initial data sample. They start with the original data and add subtle changes (called distortion), gradually making it less similar to the original. This distortion is carefully controlled to ensure that the generated data remains consistent and realistic.

After adding distortion over many iterations, the diffusion model reverses the process, where the distortion is gradually removed through an inverse de-distortion process to produce a new data sample that resembles the original sample.

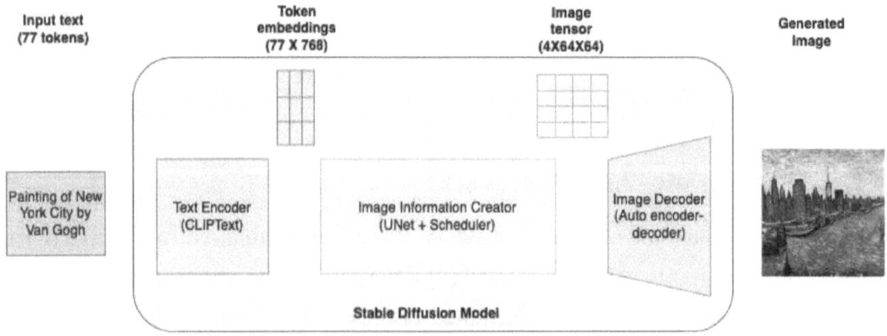

b. Generated Competitive Networks

The Generative Adversarial Network (GAN) is another generative AI model based on the concept of the diffusion model.

Generative adversarial networks work by training two neural networks competitively. The first network, known as a generator, creates false data samples by adding random distortion. The second network, called a discriminator, attempts to distinguish between real data and fake data produced by the generator.

During training, the generator continually improves its ability to generate realistic data, while the discriminator becomes better at distinguishing between real and fake data. This competitive process continues until the generator produces data so convincing that the discriminator cannot distinguish it from the real data.

Generative adversarial networks are widely used in photorealistic image generation, pattern transfer, and data augmentation tasks.

c. Variable Autoencoders

Variational autoencoders (VAE) recognize the existence of a compressed representation of data called latent space. This latent space is a mathematical representation of the data. You can think of it as a unique code that represents data based on all of its attributes. For example, when studying faces, the latent space contains numbers representing the shape of the eyes, the shape of the nose, the cheekbones, and the ears.

Variable autoencoders use two neural networks: the encoder and the decoder. The encoder's neural network maps the input data to a mean and a variable for each dimension of the latent space. It creates a random sample from a Gaussian distribution (normal distribution). This sample appears as a point in the latent space, and represents a compressed, simplified version of the input data.

The decoder's neural network takes this sample point from the latent space and reconstructs it back into data that resembles the original input data. Mathematical functions are used to measure how well the reconstructed data matches the original data.

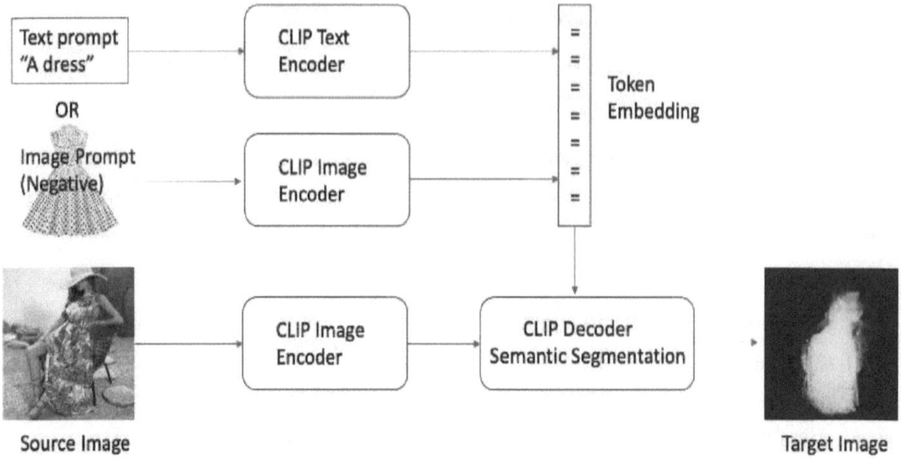

d. Transformer-Based Models

The transformer-based generative AI model is based on the concepts of encoder and decoder in the context of variable autoencoders (VAE). Transformer-based models add more layers to the encoder to improve performance on text-based tasks, such as comprehension, translation, and creative writing.

Transformer-based models use a self-attention mechanism. It evaluates the importance of different parts of the input sequence when processing each element in the sequence.

Another major advantage is that these AI models implement contextual embeddings. The encoding of a sequence element depends not only on the element itself, but also on its context within the sequence.

7.3 How Transformer-Based Models Work

To understand how transformer-based models work, imagine a sentence as a string of words.

The self-attention mechanism helps the model focus on relevant words as it processes each word. To discover different types of relationships between words, the transformer-based generative model uses multiple encoding layers called attention vertices. Each head learns to handle different parts of the input sequence. This allows the model to simultaneously consider different aspects of the data.

Each layer also refines contextual implications. Layers enhance how information-rich the embeddings are and extract everything from grammatical rules to complex semantic meanings.

7.4 How has Generative Artificial Intelligence Technology Evolved?

Elementary generative models have been used for decades in statistics to help analyze numerical data. Neural networks and deep learning were the last precursors of modern generative artificial intelligence. In 2013, Variational Autoencoders (VAE) were developed, which were the first deep generative models that could generate realistic images and speech.

These tools provided the ability to create new formats for multiple data types. This has led to the rapid emergence of other generative AI models, such as generative competitive networks and diffusion models. These innovations focused on creating data that, despite being artificially generated, increasingly closely resembles real data over time.

In 2017, another shift in AI research occurred with the advent of transformers that seamlessly integrated the architecture of encoders and decoders along with the use of a mechanism of interest. Transformers have simplified the process of training language models while achieving an exceptional level of efficiency and versatility. Prominent models, such as the Generative Pre-Trained Transformer (GPT), have emerged as foundational models that can be pre-trained on a wide range of raw texts and fine-tuned to perform various tasks.

Transformers changed what was possible for natural language processing, enabling generative capabilities to accomplish tasks ranging from translation and summarization to answering questions.

Many generative AI models continue to make great strides and have applications across multiple industries. Recent innovations focus on improving models to work on proprietary (i.e. private) data. Researchers also want to create text, images, videos and speech that are increasingly closer to what humans create.

7.5 What are the Best Practices for Adopting Generative AI?

If your organization wants to implement generative AI solutions, consider the following best practices to enhance your efforts.

a- Starting With Internal Applications

Adoption of generative AI is best started by developing internal applications, with a focus on improving operations and employee productivity. So you get a more controlled environment to test results while also building skills and understanding of the technology. You can test models extensively, and even customize them on internal knowledge sources.

This way, your customers will have a much better experience when you eventually use the templates for external applications.

b- Enhancing transparency

Make sure that communication about all applications and outputs of generative AI is clear, so users know they are interacting with AI and not people. For example, an AI can present itself as artificial intelligence, or AI-based search results can be highlighted and highlighted.

This way, users can rely on their own judgment when they interact with the content. They may also be more proactive in dealing with any inaccuracies or hidden biases that the underlying models may introduce due to the limitations of their training data.

c- Implement safety measures

Apply guardrails so that generative AI applications do not allow unauthorized and inadvertent access to sensitive data. Involve security teams from the beginning so that all aspects can be taken into account from the beginning. For example, you may have to anonymize data and remove personally identifiable information (PII) before training any models on internal data.

d- Testing on a large scale

Develop automated and manual testing processes to validate results and test all types of scenarios that the generative AI system may be exposed to. Build different groups of beta testers who try apps in different ways and document the results. The model will also continually improve through testing, and you will have more control over the results and expected responses.

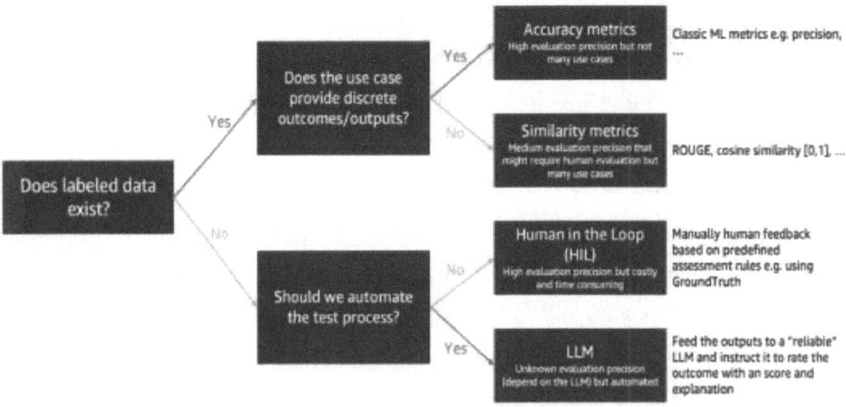

7.6 What are Common Applications of Generative AI?

With Generative AI, you can leverage machine learning to run your business more quickly and apply it to a broader range of use cases. You can apply Generative AI across all lines of business including engineering and design, marketing, customer service, finance, and sales. Code generation is one of the most promising applications of generative AI, and with Amazon Q Developer, the generative AI-powered assistant for software development, we're seeing great results on developer productivity.

Beyond generating code, there are many applications where you can apply Generative AI to bring about a step change in customer experience, employee productivity, business efficiency, and creativity. You can use Generative AI to improve customer experience with capabilities like chatbots, virtual assistants, intelligent contact centers, personalization, and content moderation. You can boost your employees' productivity with AI-powered conversational search, content creation, and text summarization among others. You can improve business processes with intelligent document processing, maintenance assistants, quality control, visual inspection, and creation of synthetic training data. Finally, you can use Generative AI to power the production of all kinds of creative content from art and music by generating text, animation, video, and images.

7.7 How Can AWS Help Generative AI?

Amazon Web Services (AWS) makes it easy to build and scale generative AI applications for your data, use cases, and customers. With Generative AI on AWS, you get enterprise-level security and privacy, access to industry-leading foundation models, applications powered by Generative AI, and a data-first approach.

Choose from a range of Generative AI services that support all types of organizations at every stage of Generative AI adoption and maturity:

Code generation (i.e. codes and icons) is one of the most promising applications of generative AI. With Amazon Q Developer, a generative AI assistant for software development, you can get great results in developer productivity.

Amazon Bedrock is another fully managed service that offers a set of high-performance foundation models and a wide range of capabilities. You can easily try out many of the best onboarding models, customize them specifically with your data, and create managed agents that execute complex business tasks.

You can also use Amazon SageMaker JumpStart to discover, explore, and deploy open source incorporation models, and even create your own. SageMaker JumpStart provides managed infrastructure and tools to accelerate the build, training, and deployment of scalable and reliable models.

AWS HealthScribe is a HIPAA-qualified service that enables healthcare software vendors to build clinical applications that automatically generate clinical notes by analyzing conversations between a patient and a physician. AWS HealthScribe combines speech recognition with generative artificial intelligence (AI) to reduce the burden of clinical documentation by transcribing patient-clinician conversations and creating clinical notes that are easier to review.

Amazon Q in QuickSight helps business analysts easily create and customize visualizations using natural language commands. New generative BI authoring capabilities extend the scope of QuickSight Q's natural language queries beyond answering questions with valid structures (such as "What are the top 10 products sold in California?") to helping analysts quickly create customizable images from question parts (such as " Top 10 Products"), and clarify the purpose of the query by asking follow-up questions, improving visuals, and completing complex calculations.

7.8 Get started with Generative AI on AWS by creating an account today

What are the current rules regarding artificial intelligence?

Governments around the world are grappling to reach an agreement regulating the use of artificial intelligence.

Recently, members of the European Parliament voted in favor of the Artificial Intelligence Law proposed by the European Union. This law - the first of its kind - will establish a strict legal framework governing the use of artificial intelligence, and companies will have to comply with it.

Margrethe Vestager says putting in place "guardrails" is essential to confront the major risks posed by artificial intelligence.

The new legislation - which is expected to come into effect in 2025 - will classify artificial intelligence applications into levels of risk - depending on their impact on consumers.

7.9 AI-powered video games and spam filters will be classified as low risk

High-risk AI applications, such as those used to assess credit scores or obtain housing, will face the strictest controls.

The United Kingdom will not adopt the application of these rules, as the British government outlined its future vision related to artificial intelligence last March.

The British government ruled out legislating a special regulatory law for artificial intelligence, and instead said that it would attach regulatory rules for artificial intelligence to the currently existing regulatory bodies that it would supervise.

But Vestager says that regulating the use of artificial intelligence should be a "global matter," and adds that adopting a "collective opinion" among "like-minded" countries is important.

During a recent hearing dedicated to artificial intelligence, US lawmakers also acknowledged concerns about the validity of these rules.

While China intends to oblige companies to notify users when using an artificial intelligence algorithm.

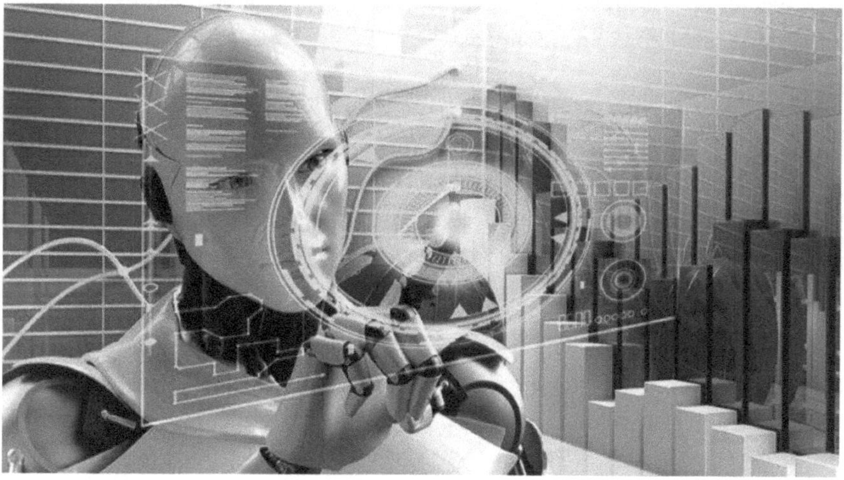

CHAPTER EIGHT

JOBS AT RISK OF EXTINCTION DUE TO ARTIFICIAL INTELLIGENCE

8.1 What Jobs are at Risk Due to Artificial Intelligence?

Artificial intelligence has great potential that will revolutionize the business world, and this raises many questions about the jobs that artificial intelligence can perform instead of humans.

A report issued by the investment bank Goldman Sachs stated that artificial intelligence could replace the equivalent of 300 million full-time jobs during the coming period, as some tasks and jobs are automated around the world.

According to the report, artificial intelligence technologies will fill a quarter of jobs in the United States and Europe.

The report highlights a number of industries and jobs that could be affected, including white-collar jobs, legal work, architecture, and management.

The report indicated that many sectors may gain huge potential benefits from the use of artificial intelligence technologies, which may ultimately lead to an increase in the total annual value of goods and services produced globally by 7 percent.

Some areas of medicine and science benefit from artificial intelligence technologies, as doctors use this technology to help detect breast cancer, and scientists use it to develop new antibiotics.

8.2 Artificial Intelligence in the Field of Intellectual Property Management

Artificial Intelligence is increasingly driving significant developments in technology and business. Artificial Intelligence is used in a wide range of industries and affects almost every aspect of creativity. The growth of artificial intelligence is fueled by the availability of large amounts of training data as well as advances in high computing power at an affordable cost. Artificial intelligence intersects with intellectual property in a number of ways.

The growth of artificial intelligence in a range of technical fields raises a number of policy questions regarding intellectual property. The main focus of these questions is whether the existing intellectual property system needs to be modified to provide balanced protection for works and innovations created by machines, artificial intelligence, and the data on which the artificial intelligence depends to function. WIPO has embarked on an open process to lead the conversation on the implications for intellectual property policy.

In the global innovation economy, the demand for intellectual property rights – patents, trademarks, industrial designs and copyright – is growing rapidly and becoming more complex. Artificial intelligence, big data analytics, and new technologies, such as blockchains, can be used to address the growing challenges facing intellectual property offices.

8.3 Artificial Intelligence in the Judiciary

The Global Judicial Integrity Network had already begun exploring the ethical use of AI in judiciaries upon its official launch in April 2018, when the Judicial Systems Research Institute organized a panel discussion on AI and court administration as one of its breakout sessions. Following this event, team member Francesco Contini subsequently wrote an article about AI based on his experience drafting the recent Council of Europe guidelines on the use of AI. His comprehensive opinion template presented on our website provides a solid overview of the issues that arise. Diana Graske of the National Center for State Courts also appeared in a podcast episode, which further describes the use of artificial intelligence to address case backlogs in judicial bodies.

In addition to these activities, the network participated in the International Conference of the Judicial Policy Research Institute of the Supreme Court of the Republic of Korea in Seoul and the United Nations Global Meeting on Data Governance and Artificial Intelligence in Geneva, where we contributed to discussions on this topic. Furthermore, the Global Judicial Integrity Network organized a panel discussion on AI as part of the World Bank's Law, Justice and Development Week in 2019, as well as at the Network's second high-level event in Doha, Qatar in 2020. The Network also recently presented on the Gender Equality Track At the ongoing Global Summit on AI for Good, participants can watch a recording of the final presentation online.

Many jurisdictions have begun using AI applications to improve efficiency. However, while AI brings with it great potential for improvement, judicial bodies must be mindful of potential challenges to ethical principles, such as transparency, accountability and impartiality when developing new projects. Of course, when using new technology, jurisdictions still need to ensure that they adhere to the Bangalore Principles.

As an emerging field, the use of AI in judicial bodies remains largely unregulated with specific guidelines and the Network hopes to draw on the experiences and good practices of its participants in the coming months to bridge this gap.

8.4 Artificial Intelligence Ethics

UNESCO, based on its unique mandate, is at the forefront of international efforts to ensure the development of science and technology in the coming decades in accordance with strong ethical standards.

Based on this vision, UNESCO has established a set of global standards, whether in the field of genetic research, climate change, or scientific research, to achieve the maximum benefit from scientific discoveries and reduce the risks of undermining them, as well as ensuring that they are harnessed to build a more comprehensive, sustainable and peaceful world. UNESCO also identified new challenges in several areas, including neurotechnology ethics, climate engineering and the Internet of Things.

The steady renaissance in artificial intelligence has created many opportunities globally, from facilitating diagnosis for healthcare purposes to enabling humans to communicate with each other through social networking sites, as well as enhancing workforce efficiency through automated tasks.

These exponential changes naturally raise serious ethical concerns stemming from the potential for artificial intelligence systems to instill bias, worsen climate degradation, threaten human rights, and much more. The risks posed by AI are already compounding existing inequalities, further harming already marginalized groups.

There is no other field that is more in need of an ethical guide than artificial intelligence. These general-purpose technologies are reshaping the way we work, interact and live. The world is changing at a pace not seen since the widespread use of the printing press six centuries ago. Artificial intelligence technologies bring great benefits in many areas. However, it is feared that in the absence of ethical controls, it will lead to the emergence of bias and discrimination on the ground, fuel divisions, and threaten human rights and fundamental freedoms.

8.5 Four Core Values

The agreement revolves around four basic values that lay the foundations for artificial intelligence systems that benefit humanity, individuals, societies, and the environment:

1-Human rights and human dignity

Respect, protect and promote human rights, fundamental freedoms and human dignity.

2-Living in peaceful societies

Fair and coherent.

3-Ensuring diversity and inclusion

4-Prosperity of the environment and ecosystems

8.6 A Vital Understanding of Artificial Intelligence

The recommendation provides an in-depth interpretation of artificial intelligence as a spectrum of systems capable of processing data in a way that simulates intelligent behavior.

Therefore, the recommendation is of great importance in view of the rapid technological change that may undermine the effectiveness of any rigid and narrow-minded definition, and hinder the implementation of precautionary policies against any future risks.

8.7 A Human Rights-Based Approach to Artificial Intelligence

There are ten key principles to lay the foundations for a human rights-based approach to AI ethics

1- Proportionality and non-harm

The use of artificial intelligence systems must not go beyond what is necessary to achieve legitimate ends. Risks must be assessed to prevent harm resulting from these uses.

2- Safety and security

Unwanted damage (safety risks) and vulnerability to attacks (security risks) must be prevented and addressed by AI actors.

3- The right to privacy and data protection

Privacy must be protected and established throughout the life cycle of AI systems. Appropriate data protection frameworks must be put in place.

4- Multiple stakeholders, adaptive governance and collaboration

International law and national sovereignty must be respected during the use of data, and diverse stakeholders must be involved to take comprehensive approaches to the governance of AI systems.

5- Responsibility and accountability

AI systems must be reviewable and agreed upon. There must be supervision and evaluation of impacts and implementation of mechanisms aimed at exercising due diligence, review and scrutiny, in order to avoid conflicts with human rights and risks that threaten environmental well-being.

6- Transparency and explainability

Deploying AI systems in an ethical manner depends on transparency and explainability. The degree of transparency and measurability must be adapted based on the context, as tense situations may arise between transparency and measurability, on the one hand, and other principles of privacy, security, and safety, on the other hand.

7- Human supervision and firmness

Member States should ensure that AI systems do not replace absolute human responsibility and accountability.

8- Sustainability

AI technologies must be evaluated based on their impacts on "sustainability" and understood as a spectrum of ever-changing goals, including the United Nations Sustainable Development Goals.

9- Awareness and literacy

Public understanding of AI and data must be enhanced through open and accessible education, civic engagement, digital skills, training in AI ethics, and media and information literacy.

10- Fairness and non-discrimination

AI actors should promote social justice, equity and non-discrimination, and take a comprehensive approach to ensure that the benefits of AI extend to all.

8.8 Activable Policies

Key policy action actions outline areas where Member States can work to take effective steps to develop AI responsibly.

There is no doubt that values and principles are truly necessary to establish the foundations of any ethical framework for artificial intelligence, but current trends regarding the ethics of artificial intelligence have emphasized the necessity of not being satisfied with high-level principles and working to find practical strategies.

This is precisely what the Recommendation provides, as it identifies 11 key areas for policy action.

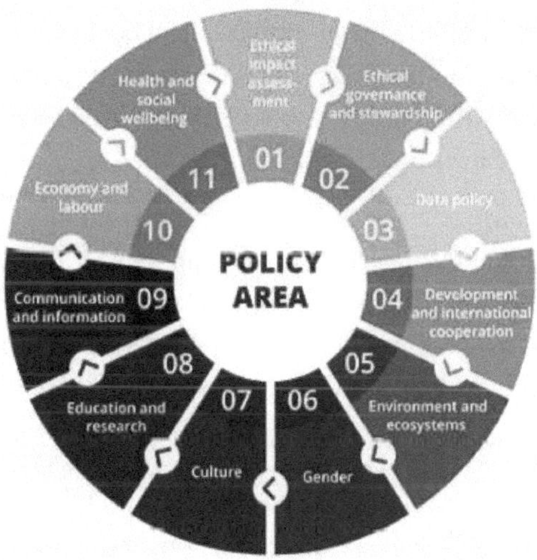
POLICY
AREA
01
Ethical impact assess-ment
02
Ethical governance and stewardship
03
Data policy
04
Development and international cooperation
05
Environment and ecosystems
06
Gender
07
Culture
08
Education and research
09
Communication and information
10
Economy and labour
11
Health and social wellbeing

8.9 Implementation of the Recommendation

There is still a long way to go to provide Member States with practical resources to ensure effective implementation of the recommendation. Therefore, UNESCO has prepared two practical methodologies:

8.10 Readiness and Preparedness Assessment Methodology

The preparedness assessment methodology is designed to assess the readiness of Member States to effectively implement the Recommendation. It helps them assess their state of preparedness and provides UNESCO with a basis for tailoring its support for capacity-building.

8.11 Ethical Impact Assessment

The EIA methodology helps AI project teams, in collaboration with affected communities, to identify and evaluate the impacts that AI systems may have, which allows identifying potential impacts and identifying precautionary measures to avoid harm.

The Women's Network for Ethical AI expert platform to advance gender equality

The Women for Ethical AI Network is a new collaborative network created by UNESCO to support efforts by governments and companies to ensure women are equally represented in the design and deployment processes of AI systems. Network members will contribute to strengthening the ethical provisions of the Convention on the Ethics of Artificial Intelligence.

The network brings together 17 leading experts from academia, civil society, the private sector and regulatory bodies around the world, who will share research and contribute to building a repertoire of good practices. The network will advance progress towards eliminating discrimination from algorithms and data sources, and stimulate the participation of girls, women and underrepresented groups in AI systems.

8.12 Ibero-American Business Council for Artificial Intelligence Ethics

The Ibero-American Business Council for Artificial Intelligence Ethics is a collaborative initiative between UNESCO and Latin American companies active in the development and use of artificial intelligence in many sectors.

The Council serves as a platform that brings together companies to share their experiences and ethical practices in the field of artificial intelligence. The Council works closely with UNESCO to ensure that artificial intelligence is developed and used in a way that respects human rights and maintains ethical standards.

Today, Microsoft and Telefonica chair the Council, which is committed to strengthening technical capabilities in the areas of ethics and artificial intelligence, designing and implementing the ethical impact assessment methodology set out in the Convention on the Ethics of Artificial Intelligence, and contributing to the development of regional smart systems. Through these efforts, the Council strives to create a competitive environment that benefits all stakeholders in Latin America and promotes responsible and ethical artificial intelligence.

8.13 Examples of ethical dilemmas

Biased Artificial Intelligence

Examples of gender-based discrimination in the context of artificial intelligence, stemming from the stereotypical representation that permeates our societies.

Artificial Intelligence in Courts of Law

Judicial systems around the world are using artificial intelligence at an increasing pace, which requires raising more ethical issues.

Artificial Intelligence Creates Arts

The use of artificial intelligence in the field of culture calls for some interesting ethical questions, such as the following question: What happens when artificial intelligence gains the ability to create works of art independently?

Self-Driving Cars

A self-driving car is a vehicle capable of sensing its surroundings and driving with little or no human intervention.

8.14 Artificial Intelligence (AI) in Cardiovascular Medicine

Utilizing artificial intelligence technologies in clinical practices

Scientists and cardiologists are collaborating to use artificial intelligence techniques to treat people with cardiovascular disease.

Mayo Clinic is at the forefront of the movement to deploy AI tools and technologies in clinical practice to help people with heart disease or those at risk for heart disease. The clinic's cardiac AI team uses these new technologies to early predict risk and diagnose complex heart problems. People who receive heart care from Mayo Clinic's Department of Cardiovascular Medicine can benefit from leading cardiology research and expertise to improve patient care.

Artificial intelligence is intelligent technologies that are automated. It touches on almost every aspect of modern life, including medicine. Artificial intelligence is used at Mayo Clinic to program computers. This aims to process and respond to data quickly and continuously in order to achieve better treatment results.

Uses of AI include detecting heart disease, treating strokes faster, and enhancing the efficiency of diagnostic radiology. For example, one Mayo Clinic study applied artificial intelligence techniques to a new screening tool for people with a certain type of heart problem that has no apparent symptoms. This condition is known as left ventricular dysfunction. This AI-powered screening tool detected people at risk for the condition in 93% of cases. To illustrate the value of this percentage, a mammogram is accurate in 85% of cases. Furthermore, AI developed by Mayo Clinic is used in Apple Watches to detect poor pumping force of the heart (reduced ventricular ejection fraction).

These techniques integrate with the knowledge that doctors have. Essentially, when combined with direct care and data analysis, AI for cardiology enables doctors to spend more time with their patients and improve shared decision-making.

8.15 Some Basics

Artificial intelligence is the ability to make computers or machines learn to solve problems that require human effort. Advances in computing power have made it easier to analyze large amounts of data quickly, consistently, and accurately. This has enabled healthcare scientists to use AI on large, complex data sets in a way that improves decision-making, diagnosis, and treatment by detecting patterns contained in patient data.

The basic unit of an AI system is a "neural network". For example, a computer system is trained by ingesting and analyzing hundreds of thousands of sets of similar reads. The computer then becomes imbued with expertise about looking at the issue being studied, such as an electrocardiogram. The result is an artificial intelligence system that can read a simple test, detect a heart condition, and predict potential problems in the future.

Mayo Clinic leaders have identified several areas that may represent an opportunity to leverage AI in the healthcare sector. Mayo Clinic is well positioned to advance the field of artificial intelligence because its long history of caring for large numbers of patients has provided it with a large database of historical genomes, microbiomes, electrocardiograms, diagnostic scan images and other test results. This is in addition to the clinic's strong culture of close collaboration between doctors, engineers and scientists, which contributes to expanding the use of artificial intelligence in healthcare in beneficial ways.

8.16 From Research to Clinical Practice

Mayo Clinic cardiovascular medicine doctors and scientists combine artificial intelligence with clinical practice for better care. Here are three examples that have moved from research to use in the clinic:

• Helping people who have had a stroke. In emergency rooms, when people have a type of stroke called intracerebral hemorrhage, they undergo CT scanning. This scan is tested using a computer trained to analyze CT data. This method has proven its ability to reduce the time taken for diagnosis and reduce brain damage.

• Avoid heart problems. The use of artificial intelligence in electrocardiography has led to the creation of low-cost tests that can be widely used to detect poor pumping power in the heart that, if left untreated, leads to heart failure. With a database of more than 7 million ECG examinations, Mayo Clinic is well-resourced to advance the field of artificial intelligence. First, all information that could identify the patient is erased to protect privacy. This data can then be researched to predict heart failure accurately and quickly.

• Early detection of atrial fibrillation. AI-guided EKG scans are used to detect arrhythmia before any symptoms appear. This arrhythmia is also called atrial fibrillation.

8.17 Collaboration that Results in Creativity

The field of artificial intelligence is witnessing rapid growth in the healthcare sector thanks to the collaborative efforts of experts. Mayo Clinic has applied methods validated in various medical and surgical specialties to improve clinical care. These groups include cardiovascular medicine, neurology, oncology, and radiology, and they share their achievements in the medical literature so that they can be widely adopted to benefit patients everywhere.

These AI tools and techniques also play an important role in education, and are used by Mayo Clinic medical students, residents, fellows and experienced surgeons to learn new or uncommon procedures. Mayo Clinic is at the forefront in this field by holding seminars on artificial intelligence in which doctors and scientists participate to develop this science in the health care sector.

8.18 Research Innovations in Cardiovascular Artificial Intelligence

The cardiovascular medicine team at Mayo Clinic is one of the leading specialties that has helped rapidly develop new AI tools and techniques and test their accuracy. Potential future uses still under development at Mayo Clinic include:

• Predicting early risks in conditions such as embolic stroke

• Monitoring the heart and detecting cardiac arrhythmias thanks to smart clothing projects

• Developing artificial intelligence technologies compatible with smartphones and high-tech hearing aids

Mayo Clinic doctors, scientists and engineers are making ongoing progress in studying and practicing artificial intelligence technologies that improve health care.

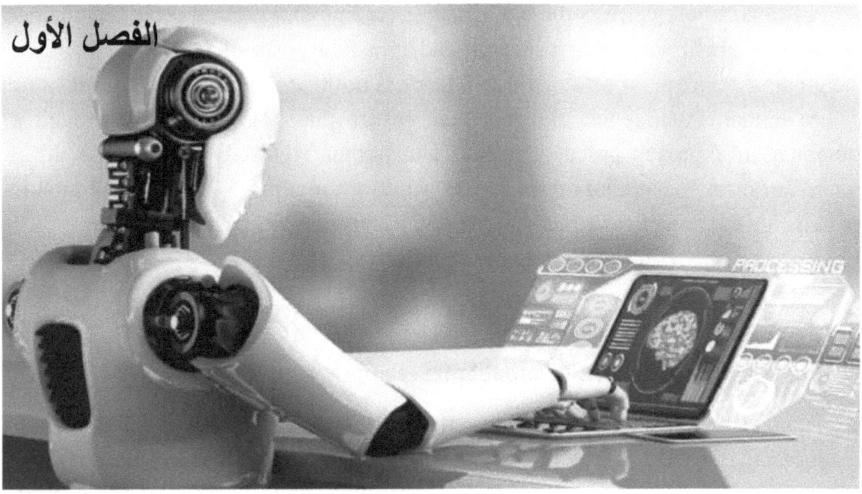

CHAPTER NINE

ETHICS OF ARTIFICIAL INTELLIGENCE

9.1 Towards the Ethics of Artificial Intelligence

We stand at the dawn of a new era. The technological revolution is changing our lives at breakneck speed, dramatically changing the ways we work, learn, and even live together. Artificial Intelligence (AI) is experiencing explosive growth and finding new applications in an increasing number of sectors, including security, environment, research, education, health, culture, and commerce along with the increasingly complex use of big data.

Artificial intelligence is the new frontier for humanity. Once these boundaries are crossed, artificial intelligence will lead to a new form of human civilization. The guiding principle of artificial intelligence is not that it becomes independent or replace human intelligence. But we must ensure that it is developed through a humanitarian approach based on values and human rights. We are faced with a crucial question: What kind of society do we want tomorrow? The AI revolution is opening up exciting new frontiers, but the anthropological and social turmoil it brings in its wake requires careful consideration.

9.2 Huge Opportunity for Sustainable Development

Transformations arising from the technological revolution, especially from developments in artificial intelligence, are relevant to every aspect of the mandate of the United Nations Educational, Scientific and Cultural Organization (UNESCO). Education is already being profoundly advanced by AI. The tools of education—the way we learn, obtain knowledge, and train teachers—will not soon be the same. From now on, digital skills acquisition stands at the heart of all our educational programmes. Moreover, we must "learn to learn" as the speed of innovation is rapidly changing the labor market. Today, more than ever, the humanities such as history, philosophy and literature are crucial to our ability to function in our rapidly changing world. Artificial intelligence in the field of culture is already being widely used. For example, in photographs used to reconstruct heritage. It is used in science as well, especially in our environmental programs and underwater research. Communications and information also depend directly on advances in artificial intelligence, especially with regard to freedom of expression and access to information.

Artificial Intelligence can open huge opportunities to achieve the Sustainable Development Goals (SDGs) set by the United Nations in the 2030 Agenda for Sustainable Development. Its applications enable innovative solutions, improved risk assessment, better planning and faster knowledge sharing.

9.3 Addressing Artificial Intelligence Challenges

While AI represents an incredible asset for responsible development in our societies, it also raises major ethical issues. How can we ensure that algorithms do not violate basic human rights from privacy and data confidentiality to freedom of choice and freedom of conscience? Can freedom of action be guaranteed when our desires are predictable and directed? How can we ensure that social and cultural stereotypes are not replicated in AI software, especially when it comes to gender discrimination? Can these circuits be repeated? Can values be programmed, and by whom? How can we ensure accountability when decisions and actions are fully automated? How do we make sure that no one, wherever they are in the world, is deprived of the benefits of these technologies? How can we ensure that AI is developed in a transparent way so that global citizens whose lives are affected have a say in its development?

To answer these questions, we must distinguish between the direct impacts of artificial intelligence on our societies, its consequences that we are already feeling, and its long-term repercussions. This requires that we collectively form a vision and strategic action plan.

9.4 Establishing a Global Dialogue on the Ethics of Artificial Intelligence:

The world must ensure that new technologies, especially those based on artificial intelligence, are used for the benefit of our societies and their sustainable development. AI developments and applications must be regulated so that they are compatible with the fundamental rights that shape our democratic horizon.

Many actors such as companies, research centers, academies of sciences, UN member states, international organizations and civil society associations are calling for an ethical framework for the development of artificial intelligence. While understanding of the issues is increasing, related initiatives need more robust coordination. This problem is global, and must be thought about at a global level to avoid a "pick and choose" approach to ethics. Moreover, a comprehensive and global approach, with the participation of UN funds, agencies and programmes, is required if we are to find ways to harness artificial intelligence for sustainable development.

UNESCO will be a full and active participant in this global conversation. Our organization has many years of experience in science and technology ethics. Our advisory bodies have already issued several reports and declarations, including on robotics, such as the report of the Global Commission on the Ethics of Scientific Knowledge and Technology on the ethics of robots in 2017. The advisory bodies also have experience in developing normative tools, including the Universal

Declaration on the Human Genome and Human Rights Human Rights in 1997 and the Universal Declaration on Bioethics and Human Rights in 2005.

UNESCO's priorities should also guide our international work in this area. It is essential to ensure that Africa fully participates in AI-related transformations, not only as a beneficiary but also as an upstream participant, contributing directly to its development. Regarding gender equality, we must combat biases in our societies to ensure they are not replicated in AI applications. Finally, we must empower young people by equipping them with the skills they need for life in the 21st century to integrate into the changing labor market.

UNESCO is also playing a key role in bridging existing gaps that AI is likely to deepen. Eliminating fragmentation across countries and genders, as well as in terms of resources and knowledge, will enable more people to contribute to the ongoing digital transformation.

UNESCO, with its humanitarian mission and international dimension, bringing together researchers, philosophers, programmers, policymakers, representatives of the private sector and civil society, is the natural venue for debate on these ethical issues. UNESCO will organize discussions on AI in several regions of the world starting late this year, bringing together experts from a wide range of backgrounds and experiences. The first discussion, which took place in Marrakesh, Morocco, on December 12, 2018, focused on artificial intelligence and Africa. A second international conference was held at UNESCO headquarters in Paris in the first half of 2019. These conferences could eventually lead to a dialogue, with the agreement of Member States, to define key ethical principles to accompany developments in the field of artificial intelligence.

As a global forum where everyone's voice is heard and respected, UNESCO is fulfilling its role, enlightening global debate on the major transformations of our time while setting principles to ensure that technological progress is used for the common good. The promise of AI and the ethical issues inherent in it are remarkable, and our responses to these challenges will change our image of the world.

Together we must find the best solutions to ensure that the development of artificial intelligence is an opportunity for humanity, as our generation has the responsibility to transition to a more just, peaceful and prosperous society.

9.5 Seven Ways Artificial Intelligence Will Change Nuclear Science and Technology

Over the past decade, artificial intelligence has witnessed rapid development and has become capable of solving the most complex problems, and it is used in various sectors such as industry, transportation, finance, education, and health care. The popularity of artificial intelligence is increasing in the Arab world, according to the Arab American Organization. In Saudi Arabia, artificial intelligence is a major goal of the Kingdom's Vision 2030, which will include reforms in the areas of infrastructure, health care, and education to improve citizens' conditions. The United Arab Emirates is one of the Arab countries that invests in artificial intelligence. It even laid the foundation stone for the Ministry of Artificial Intelligence in 2017, and launched the "Emirates Artificial Intelligence Strategy" initiative, which includes several sectors, including transportation, health, space, energy, technology, and education.

Likewise, artificial intelligence has the potential to advance the development of nuclear applications and science and technology. Harnessing the capabilities of artificial intelligence in the nuclear field can have a positive impact on addressing some of today's most pressing challenges, from food security to climate change.

Here are some ways in which artificial intelligence will continue to benefit peaceful applications of nuclear technology. These methods are discussed in detail in a new International Atomic Energy Agency (IAEA) publication, Using Artificial Intelligence to Advance Nuclear Science and Technology Applications.

1. Human health

Artificial Intelligence contributes to the fight against diseases, as its applications are already being used to support cancer diagnosis and treatment by improving image interpretation and accurately mapping tumor contours. This allows for more precise treatment plans and adaptive radiotherapy, a process tailored to the anatomical features of each individual patient.

Artificial intelligence will also play an important role in the Agency's Zoonotic Disease Integrated Action (ZODIC) initiative to help experts better understand the impact of zoonotic diseases on human health, as well as anticipate, assess and contain future outbreaks of such diseases.

2. Food and agriculture

Artificial intelligence tools combined with nuclear technology can help make food systems more sustainable and resilient to climate change, while also addressing food and nutrition insecurity.

Experts use artificial intelligence to process and analyze data to increase crop yields, estimate soil moisture, reclaim radioactively contaminated land, detect and predict food fraud and improve irrigation.

3. Water and environment

Using isotopic methods, experts can study and track how water moves through different phases of the hydrological cycle as well as the shifts that occur in this cycle due to climate change. Experts are already applying AI-based approaches to rapidly analyze vast amounts of water-related isotope data stored in global repositories, such as the Global Precipitation Isotope Network maintained by the Agency and the World Meteorological Organization.

Thanks to the effective analysis of data easily obtained by artificial intelligence, scientists can understand climate change and its impact on water availability around the world.

4. Nuclear science and fusion research

Artificial intelligence plays an increasingly important role in nuclear science. It is used in data analysis, theoretical modeling and experimental design, helping to accelerate basic research, for example in the field of evaluating and compiling nuclear and atomic data, and promoting technological innovation.

Fusion research is one area that particularly benefits from the application of artificial intelligence. With its ability to find solutions to large and complex problems, artificial intelligence can aid scientific experiments and discoveries through modeling and simulations. These artificial intelligence applications are included in a coordinated five-year IAEA research project aimed at accelerating the pace of research and development in the field of nuclear fusion.

5. Nuclear powers

Nuclear power is a reliable, low-carbon source of energy, and could greatly benefit from the inclusion of artificial intelligence. By combining digital simulations of real nuclear facilities with artificial intelligence systems, the field can simplify complex procedures and improve reactor design, performance and safety. This improvement can increase process efficiency and reduce maintenance costs.

Machine learning, a process through which artificial intelligence learns to analyze massive amounts of data, helps automate tasks and thus increase reliability and avoid errors. In addition, AI has significant analytical and predictive potential to help monitor nuclear power plant operations and detect anomalies.

6. Nuclear security and radiation protection

As more countries move toward harnessing nuclear technology for peaceful uses and adopt nuclear power programs, the Agency is continuously working to ensure that people and the environment are protected from the potentially harmful effects of ionizing radiation.

Artificial intelligence can contribute to nuclear safety and security in several ways. It can be used to process data extracted from radiation detection systems to enhance the detection and identification of nuclear and other radioactive materials. Artificial intelligence can be used to analyze data extracted from physical security systems to improve intruder detection. AI can also help identify anomalies that could indicate a cyberattack on a nuclear facility. Moreover, in the field of radiation protection, the integration of artificial intelligence into programs related to safety standards can enhance the protection of millions of workers occupationally exposed to radiation in the fields of medicine, construction, mining, shipping, agriculture and nuclear power.

7. Guarantees

Safeguards are technical verification measures through which the Agency provides assurances that states are respecting their legal obligations to use nuclear materials only for peaceful purposes. The IAEA assesses declared nuclear material and related activities by States and seeks to verify the absence of undeclared nuclear material by imposing certain measures, such as inspections at nuclear facilities and sites.

The safeguards rely on vast amounts of data obtained through a variety of means, such as satellite imagery, environmental sampling, gamma spectroscopy, and video monitoring. Artificial intelligence can help inspectors and safeguards analysts analyze this data. Machine learning methods are already being used to spot outliers in large data sets, help verify spent fuel, and analyze monitoring recordings. It is expected that artificial intelligence will continue to improve the efficiency of safeguards implementation by reducing repetitive tasks undertaken by inspectors.

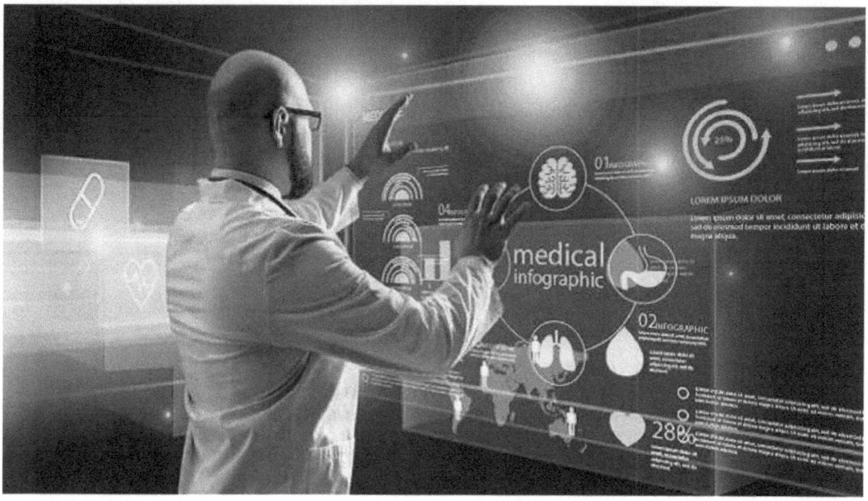

CHAPTER TEN

FUTURE PROSPECTS

10.1 Future prospects

The IAEA provides multidisciplinary forums for professionals to discuss and promote collaboration on the use of AI in applications, nuclear science and technology, and is committed to sharing knowledge and establishing partnerships via the AI for Atom platform. As part of the initiative, the agency is collaborating with the International Telecommunication Union, the UN Inter-Agency Working Group on Artificial Intelligence and nearly 40 other UN organizations to provide a solid foundation for accelerating sustainable development through artificial intelligence.

10.2 Artificial Intelligence Tools and Applications at WIPO

The Center for Advanced Technology Applications at the World Intellectual Property Organization (WIPO) develops and makes available a range of AI-powered services and tools to assist users and stakeholders. These services leverage the power of artificial intelligence to enhance efficiency, accuracy and accessibility in various areas of intellectual property.

Some notable services provided by the center include:

WIPO speech-to-text tool

WIPO Speech-to-Text is a service that converts spoken language into written text shortly after a meeting. This technology is particularly important in the context of meetings, where an accurate transcript must be prepared in a timely manner. WIPO's speech-to-text tool helps users understand and access the content of discussions and deliberations more efficiently.

WIPO Translate tool

WIPO Translate is a service provided by WIPO for advanced machine translation. This tool uses neural network technologies to provide machine translation of patent documents, scientific articles, and other intellectual property-related content. The tool supports multiple language pairs and helps users overcome language barriers and facilitate global knowledge sharing and understanding.

Automated patent classification

The Center for Advanced Technology Applications has developed an artificial intelligence-based system for automated patent classification. This system uses advanced machine learning algorithms to classify patent documents in specific technology areas, for example, using the International Patent Classification system.

Automated patent classification helps simplify patent examination procedures, improves search accuracy, and facilitates retrieval of relevant patent information.

Search Based on Similar Images Within the Global Tag Database

The Global Tag Database, maintained by WIPO, enables searches based on similar images using artificial intelligence. This tool allows users to upload images or logos and find similar or matching brands in the database. This service helps trademark professionals and trademark owners identify potential trademark infringements and conduct searches to ensure that the trademark is not being used.

Vienna Classification Assistant

The Vienna Classification Assistant is an artificial intelligence-based tool developed by WIPO to support the use of the Vienna Classification System. This system helps to classify the figurative elements of trademarks by automatically suggesting appropriate Vienna Classification symbols. The Vienna Classification Assistant enhances the accuracy and efficiency of trademark classification processes.

Automated Sorting of Internal Training Applications

WIPO's Advanced Technology Applications Center also uses artificial intelligence to automate the screening and processing of internship applications. This artificial intelligence-based system helps sort and manage a large number of internship applications effectively, ensuring the integrity and simplicity of the selection process.

The Search is Based on Similar Images Within the Global Database of Designs

WIPO's Advanced Technology Applications Center is developing similar image-based search capabilities in the global design database. This future feature will enable users to upload images of designs and find visually similar designs, facilitate design searches, and help protect industrial designs.

Description of Pictures:

The Advanced Technology Applications Center is developing a new tool that will enable users to generate keywords that will facilitate the search for similar brands and help users fill out the required descriptions.

System for Searching for Goods and Services

WIPO is developing a goods and services search system that will leverage artificial intelligence technologies to enhance the accuracy and efficiency of searching for goods and services in trademark databases. It will help users evaluate the use and accuracy of descriptions of goods and services. This system also aims to improve the classification and identification processes for goods and services associated with trademarks.

10.3 Top 10 Challenges Facing AI in the Near Future

2024 is expected to witness an unprecedented boom in the development of artificial intelligence, redefining human-machine interactions, but it tends to face challenges in meeting ethical obligations.

As the risk of data security and privacy breaches increases with the spread of artificial intelligence, requiring stronger regulations and frameworks to protect sensitive information.

AI also raises concerns about job losses and the ongoing challenges of economic inequality, which calls for steps to reskill the workforce and address social and economic disparities.

1- Bias in AI

Bias in AI can be defined as the ability of machine learning algorithms to replicate and amplify pre-existing biases in the training dataset.

This can lead to unfair and unethical outcomes, which greatly impacts marginalized communities.

For example, biased hiring procedures, loan approvals, and unequal criminal sentences.

Mitigating AI bias requires a thoughtful approach to data selection, preprocessing techniques, and algorithm design to minimize bias and promote fairness.

Continuous monitoring and evaluation of AI systems also helps identify and correct bias.

Thus, fairness is promoted through AI-based decision-making processes.

2- Ethical Issues

Ethics in AI involves discussions on various issues, including privacy violations, perpetuating bias, and social impact.

Accountability, transparency, and fairness in the decisions made by AI systems are becoming the biggest challenge of the moment.

In addition, a more focused approach should be used when implementing AI in sensitive areas such as health and criminal justice that call for greater consideration of the ethical principles necessary to achieve fair outcomes.

Finding a balance between technological development and ethical issues is essential to using AI for societal benefit while avoiding risks and encouraging ethical innovation.

3- AI Integration

AI integration means integrating AI systems into production and services to improve automation and efficiency.

This means identifying relevant application scenarios, tuning AI models for specific scenarios, and ensuring compatibility with existing systems.

The integration process requires AI experts and domain specialists to work together to refine their solutions to meet regulatory requirements.

Challenges include data interoperability, the need for employee training, and associated change management.

Addressing these challenges requires strategic planning, stakeholder engagement, and iterative implementation to optimize AI and minimize disruption.

As such, AI integration can play a critical role in driving transformational change and delivering competitive advantage across industries and sectors.

4- Data Privacy and Integrity

Data security and privacy are key issues because AI systems require large amounts of data to operate and train.

To avoid leaks, breaches, and misuse, one must ensure the security, availability, and integrity of data.

Therefore, building trust among users through transparent data processes and ethical data handling protocols is critical to user confidence in AI systems and responsible data management.

5- Legal Issues Related to AI

Legal concerns around AI cover a wide spectrum, including liability, intellectual property rights, and regulatory compliance.

Legal issues related to copyright arise due to ownership of AI-generated content and algorithms.

Furthermore, regulatory regimes, which are usually the last to adapt to technological changes, must be observed to avoid legal liabilities and risks.

Addressing these issues requires a combination of legal professionals, policymakers, and technology experts working together to develop clear rules and policies that balance innovation and accountability and protect the rights of stakeholders.

6- AI Transparency

Transparency is essential to building credibility, trust, accountability, and user confidence in AI systems.

Transparency is defined as an element of how AI models work and what AI models do, including inputs, outputs, and underlying logic.

Techniques such as explainable AI aim to provide understandable insights into complex AI systems, making them easy to understand.

Moreover, clear documentation of data sources, model training methodologies, and performance metrics can also enhance transparency.

7- Software Downtime

Downtime in AI software poses significant risks, including erroneous outputs, system failures, or cyberattacks.

Testing and quality assurance practices must be rigorous at every stage of the software lifecycle to eliminate these risks.

In addition, implementing robust error handling mechanisms and contingency plans helps keep the impact of downtime small when it does occur.

Regular software updates and maintenance are also important in preventing potential defects that could cause malfunction.

In addition, creating a culture that promotes transparency and accountability helps in discovering and resolving software issues more quickly, which contributes to the reliability and safety of AI systems.

8- Limited knowledge of AI

Limited knowledge among the general population is one of the critical issues that impact informed decision-making, adoption, and regulation.

Misconceptions and misinterpretations of AI capabilities and limitations are multiplying, hindering its responsible use and promotion.

Effective measures for education and public awareness programs must be developed and implemented to ensure general understanding of AI concepts, use cases, and potential impacts.

Furthermore, enabling accessible resources and training opportunities will enable users to use AI technology more effectively.

9- Building trust

Trust in AI systems is an important condition for their widespread use and acceptance by the public.

The foundation of trust is transparency, trustworthiness, and accountability. Organizations need to ensure transparency by disclosing how AI systems work and their options.

Trustworthiness is another way of saying that you are expected to deliver consistent performance, including delivering correct results.

Accountability involves taking responsibility for the outcomes of AI, as well as correcting errors or biases.

Furthermore, building trust involves communicating with stakeholders, taking feedback, and putting ethics at the forefront.

By emphasizing transparency, trustworthiness, and accountability, organizations will build trust in AI systems, allowing users to embrace AI technologies and their potential benefits.

10. High Expectations

High expectations about AI capabilities often lead to unrealistic expectations, followed by disappointment.

While AI offers tremendous potential, its limitations and complexities often overshadow its overblown promises.

Furthermore, educational and awareness programs give stakeholders a clear picture of how AI is used and its limitations.

By setting achievable goals and having a balanced understanding of the pros and cons of AI, organizations avoid disappointment and focus on leveraging AI.

REFERENCES

1. S. Minaee *et al.*, "Large Language Models: A Survey." arXiv, Feb. 09, 2024. doi: 10.48550/arXiv.2402.06196.
2. J. Wei *et al.*, "Emergent Abilities of Large Language Models." arXiv, Oct. 26, 2022. doi: 10.48550/arXiv.2206.07682.
3. E. Seger *et al.*, "Open-Sourcing Highly Capable Foundation Models: An evaluation of risks, benefits, and alternative methods for pursuing open-source objectives." arXiv, Sep. 29, 2023. doi: 10.48550/arXiv.2311.09227.
4. E. Hubinger *et al.*, "Sleeper Agents: Training Deceptive LLMs that Persist Through Safety Training." arXiv, Jan. 17, 2024. doi: 10.48550/arXiv.2401.05566.
5. Frank Lucas, Zoe Lofgren, Mike Collins, Haley Stevens, Jay Olbernolte, and Valerie Foushee, "Letter to Dr. Laurie Locascio," Dec. 14, 2023. Available: https://republicans-science.house.gov/_cache/files/8/a/8a9f893d-858a-419f-9904-52163f22be71/191E586AF744B32E6831A248CD7F4D41.2023-12-14-aisi-scientific-merit-final-signed.pdf
6. S. Fitch, "Emergent Abilities in Large Language Models: An Explainer," Center for Security and Emerging Technology. Available: https://cset.georgetown.edu/article/emergent-abilities-in-large-language-models-an-explainer/
7. "emergence." Available: https://dictionary.cambridge.org/us/dictionary/english/emergence
8. "Emergence," *Wikipedia*. Apr. 28, 2024. Available: https://en.wikipedia.org/w/index.php?title=Emergence&oldid=1221163474
9. D. Hendrycks, N. Carlini, J. Schulman, and J. Steinhardt, "Unsolved Problems in ML Safety," *ArXiv*, Sep. 2021, Available: https://www.semanticscholar.org/paper/Unsolved-Problems-in-ML-Safety-Hendrycks-Carlini/05c2e1ee203be217f100d2da05bdcc52004f00b6?sort=is-influential
10. T. B. Brown *et al.*, "Language Models are Few-Shot Learners." arXiv, Jul. 22, 2020. Available: http://arxiv.org/abs/2005.14165
11. M. Caron *et al.*, "Emerging Properties in Self-Supervised Vision Transformers," *2021 IEEECVF Int. Conf. Comput. Vis. ICCV*, pp. 9630–9640, Oct. 2021, doi: 10.1109/ICCV48922.2021.00951.
12. "Future ML Systems Will Be Qualitatively Different," Bounded Regret. Available: https://bounded-regret.ghost.io/future-ml-systems-will-be-qualitatively-different/
13. R. Bommasani *et al.*, "On the Opportunities and Risks of Foundation Models." arXiv, Jul. 12, 2022. doi: 10.48550/arXiv.2108.07258.

14. P. W. Anderson, "More Is Different," *Science*, vol. 177, no. 4047, pp. 393–396, Aug. 1972, doi: 10.1126/science.177.4047.393.
    A. Srivastava *et al.*, "Beyond the Imitation Game: Quantifying and extrapolating the capabilities of language models." arXiv, Jun. 12, 2023. doi: 10.48550/arXiv.2206.04615.
15. R. Schaeffer, B. Miranda, and S. Koyejo, "Are Emergent Abilities of Large Language Models a Mirage?" arXiv, May 22, 2023. doi: 10.48550/arXiv.2304.15004.
16. S. Lu, I. Bigoulaeva, R. Sachdeva, H. T. Madabushi, and I. Gurevych, "Are Emergent Abilities in Large Language Models just In-Context Learning?" arXiv, Sep. 04, 2023. doi: 10.48550/arXiv.2309.01809.
17. S. Bubeck *et al.*, "Sparks of Artificial General Intelligence: Early experiments with GPT-4." arXiv, Apr. 13, 2023. doi: 10.48550/arXiv.2303.12712.
18. "The Calculi of Emergence: Computation, Dynamics, and Induction." Available: https://csc.ucdavis.edu/~cmg/compmech/pubs/CalcEmergTitlePage.htm
19. L. Saitta and M. Sebag, "Phase Transitions in Machine Learning," in *Encyclopedia of Machine Learning*, C. Sammut and G. I. Webb, Eds., Boston, MA: Springer US, 2010, pp. 767–773. doi: 10.1007/978-0-387-30164-8_635.
20. H. Cui, F. Behrens, F. Krzakala, and L. Zdeborová, "A phase transition between positional and semantic learning in a solvable model of dot-product attention." arXiv, Feb. 06, 2024. doi: 10.48550/arXiv.2402.03902.
21. *Heaven, Will Douglas (16 November 2023). "Google DeepMind wants to define what counts as artificial general intelligence". MIT Technology Review. Retrieved 1 March 2024.*
22. *Krishna, Sri (9 February 2023). "What is artificial narrow intelligence (ANI)?". VentureBeat. Retrieved 1 March 2024.*
23. *"OpenAI Charter". openai.com. Retrieved 6 April 2023.*
24. *Heath, Alex (18 January 2024). "Mark Zuckerberg's new goal is creating artificial general intelligence". The Verge. Retrieved 13 June 2024.*
25. *Baum, Seth, A Survey of Artificial General Intelligence Projects for Ethics, Risk, and Policy (PDF), Global Catastrophic Risk Institute Working Paper 20, archived (PDF) from the original on 14 November 2021, retrieved 13 January 2022*
26. Jump up to:[a b c] *"AI timelines: What do experts in artificial intelligence expect for the future?". Our World in Data. Retrieved 6 April 2023.*
27. *"Microsoft Researchers Claim GPT-4 Is Showing "Sparks" of AGI". Futurism. Retrieved 13 December 2023.*
28. *Morozov, Evgeny (30 June 2023). "The True Threat of Artificial Intelligence". The New York Times. Archived from the original on 30 June 2023. Retrieved 30 June 2023.*
29. *"Impressed by artificial intelligence? Experts say AGI is coming next, and it has 'existential' risks". ABC News. 23 March 2023. Retrieved 6 April 2023.*

30. "Artificial general intelligence: Are we close, and does it even make sense to try?". MIT Technology Review. Retrieved 6 April 2023.
31. "What is artificial superintelligence (ASI)? | Definition from TechTarget". Enterprise AI. Retrieved 8 October 2023.
32. "Artificial intelligence is transforming our world – it is on all of us to make sure that it goes well". Our World in Data. Retrieved 8 October 2023.
33. Dickson, Ben (16 November 2023). "Here is how far we are to achieving AGI, according to DeepMind". VentureBeat.
34. "Eugene Goostman is a real boy – the Turing Test says so". The Guardian. 9 June 2014. ISSN 0261-3077. Retrieved 3 March 2024.
35. Varanasi, Lakshmi (21 March 2023). "AI models like ChatGPT and GPT-4 are acing everything from the bar exam to AP Biology. Here's a list of difficult exams both AI versions have passed". Business Insider. Retrieved 30 May 2023.
36. Naysmith, Caleb (7 February 2023). "6 Jobs Artificial Intelligence Is Already Replacing and How Investors Can Capitalize on It". Retrieved 30 May 2023.
37. Turk, Victoria (28 January 2015). "The Plan to Replace the Turing Test with a 'Turing Olympics'". Vice. Retrieved 3 March 2024.
38. Gopani, Avi (25 May 2022). "Turing Test is unreliable. The Winograd Schema is obsolete. Coffee is the answer". Analytics India Magazine. Retrieved 3 March 2024.
39. Bhaimiya, Sawdah (20 June 2023). "DeepMind's co-founder suggested testing an AI chatbot's ability to turn $100,000 into $1 million to measure human-like intelligence". Business Insider. Retrieved 3 March 2024.
40. Suleyman, Mustafa (14 July 2023). "Mustafa Suleyman: My new Turing test would see if AI can make $1 million". MIT Technology Review. Retrieved 3 March 2024.
41. "AI Index: State of AI in 13 Charts". Stanford University Human-Centered Artificial Intelligence. 15 April 2024. Retrieved 27 May 2024.
42. Kaplan, Andreas (2022). "Artificial Intelligence, Business and Civilization – Our Fate Made in Machines". Archived from the original on 6 May 2022. Retrieved 12 March 2022.
43. Jump up to:[a] [b] Hutter, Marcus (2005). Universal Artificial Intelligence: Sequential Decisions Based on Algorithmic Probability. Texts in Theoretical Computer Science an EATCS Series. Springer. doi:10.1007/b138233. ISBN 978-3-540-26877-2. S2CID 33352850. Archived from the original on 19 July 2022. Retrieved 19 July 2022.
44. Legg, Shane (2008). Machine Super Intelligence (PDF) (Thesis). University of Lugano. Archived (PDF) from the original on 15 June 2022. Retrieved 19 July 2022.
45. "Избираеми дисциплини 2010/2011 – зимен триместър" [Elective courses 2010/2011 – winter trimester]. Факултет по математика и информатика [Faculty of Mathematics and Informatics] (in Bulgarian). Archived from the original on 26 July 2020. Retrieved 11 May 2020.

46. *Shevlin, Henry; Vold, Karina; Crosby, Matthew; Halina, Marta (4 October 2019). "The limits of machine intelligence: Despite progress in machine intelligence, artificial general intelligence is still a major challenge". EMBO Reports. **20** (10): e49177. doi:10.15252/embr.201949177. ISSN 1469-221X. PMC 6776890. PMID 31531926.*
47. *Bubeck, Sébastien; Chandrasekaran, Varun; Eldan, Ronen; Gehrke, Johannes; Horvitz, Eric; Kamar, Ece; Lee, Peter; Lee, Yin Tat; Li, Yuanzhi; Lundberg, Scott; Nori, Harsha; Palangi, Hamid; Ribeiro, Marco Tulio; Zhang, Yi (27 March 2023). "Sparks of Artificial General Intelligence: Early experiments with GPT-4". arXiv:2303.12712 [cs.CL].*
48. *Boucher, Philip (March 2019). "Concluding remarks". How artificial intelligence works (PDF) (Report). European Parliamentary Research Service. Archived (PDF) from the original on 3 March 2020. Retrieved 3 March 2020. Today's AI is powerful and useful, but remains far from speculated AGI or ASI.*
49. itu.int: Beyond Mad?: The Race For Artificial General Intelligence Archived 9 ovember 2020 at the Wayback Machine, "AGI represents a level of power that remains firmly in the realm of speculative fiction as on date." February 2, 2018, retrieved March 3, 2020
50. *Deane, George (2022). "Machines That Feel and Think: The Role of Affective Feelings and Mental Action in (Artificial) General Intelligence". Artificial Life. **28** (3): 289–309. doi:10.1162/artl_a_00368. ISSN 1064-5462. PMID 35881678. S2CID 251069071.*
51. *Fjelland, Ragnar (17 June 2020). "Why general artificial intelligence will not be ealized". Humanities and Social Sciences Communications. 7 (1): 1–9. doi:10.1057/s41599-020-0494-4. hdl:11250/2726984. ISSN 2662-9992. S2CID 219710554.*
52. *Khatchadourian, Raffi (23 November 2015). "The Doomsday Invention: Will artificial intelligence bring us utopia or destruction?". The New Yorker. Archived from the original on 28 January 2016. Retrieved 7 February 2016.*
53. *"Microsoft Now Claims GPT-4 Shows 'Sparks' of General Intelligence". 24 March 2023.*
54. *Shimek, Cary (6 July 2023). "AI Outperforms Humans in Creativity est". Neuroscience News. Retrieved 20 October 2023.*
55. *Guzik, Erik E.; Byrge, Christian; Gilde, Christian (1 December 2023). "The originality of machines: AI takes the Torrance Test". Journal of Creativity. **33** (3): 100065. doi:10.1016/j.yjoc.2023.100065. ISSN 2713-3745. S2CID 261087185.*
56. *Zia, Tehseen (8 January 2024). "Unveiling of Large Multimodal Models: Shaping the Landscape of Language Models in 2024". Unite.ai. Retrieved 26 May 2024.*
57. *"AI Index: State of AI in 13 Charts". hai.stanford.edu. 15 April 2024. Retrieved 7 June 2024.*

58. *"Next-Gen AI: OpenAI and Meta's Leap Towards Reasoning Machines". Unite.ai. 19 April 2024. Retrieved 7 June 2024.*

59. *James, Alex P. (2022). "The Why, What, and How of Artificial General Intelligence Chip Development". IEEE Transactions on Cognitive and Developmental Systems. **14** (2): 333–347. arXiv:2012.06338. doi:10.1109/TCDS.2021.3069871. ISSN 2379-8920. S2CID 228376556. Archived from the original on 28 August 2022. Retrieved 28 August 2022.*

60. *Pei, Jing; Deng, Lei; Song, Sen; Zhao, Mingguo; Zhang, Youhui; Wu, Shuang; Wang, Guanrui; Zou, Zhe; Wu, Zhenzhi; He, Wei; Chen, Feng; Deng, Ning; Wu, Si; Wang, Yu; Wu, Yujie (2019). "Towards artificial general intelligence with hybrid Tianjic chip architecture". Nature. **572** (7767):111. Bibcode:2019Natur.572..106P. doi:10.1038/s41586-019-1424-8. ISSN 1476-4687. PMID 31367028. S2CID 199056116. Archived from the original on 29 August 2022. Retrieved 29 August 2022.*

61. *Pandey, Mohit; Fernandez, Michael; Gentile, Francesco; Isayev, Olexandr; Tropsha, Alexander; Stern, Abraham C.; Cherkasov, Artem (March 2022). "The transformational role of GPU computing and deep learning in drug discovery". Nature Machine Intelligence. **4** (3): 211–221. doi:10.1038/s42256-022-00463-x. ISSN 2522-5839. S2CID 252081559.*

62. *Liu, Feng; Shi, Yong; Liu, Ying (2017). "Intelligence Quotient and Intelligence Grade of Artificial Intelligence". Annals of Data Science. **4** (2): 179–191. arXiv:1709.10242. doi:10.1007/s40745-017-0109-0. S2CID 37900130.*

63. *Brien, Jörn (5 October 2017). "Google-KI doppelt so schlau wie Siri" [Google AI is twice as smart as Siri – but a six-year-old beats both] (in German). Archived from the original on 3 January 2019. Retrieved 2 January 2019.*

64. *Grossman, Gary (3 September 2020). "We're entering the AI twilight zone between narrow and general AI". VentureBeat. Archived from the original on 4 September 2020. Retrieved 5 September 2020. Certainly, too, there are those who claim we are already seeing an early example of an AGI system in the recently announced GPT-3 natural language processing (NLP) neural network. ... So is GPT-3 the first example of an AGI system? This is debatable, but the consensus is that it is not AGI. ... If nothing else, GPT-3 tells us there is a middle ground between narrow and general AI.*

65. *Quach, Katyanna. "A developer built an AI chatbot using GPT-3 that helped a man speak again to his late fiancée. OpenAI shut it down". The Register. Archived from the original on 16 October 2021. Retrieved 16 October 2021.*

66. *Wiggers, Kyle (13 May 2022), "DeepMind's new AI can perform over 600 tasks, from playing games to controlling robots", TechCrunch, archived from the original on 16 June 2022, retrieved 12 June 2022*
67. *Bubeck, Sébastien; Chandrasekaran, Varun; Eldan, Ronen; Gehrke, Johannes; Horvitz, Eric; Kamar, Ece; Lee, Peter; Lee, Yin Tat; Li, Yuanzhi; Lundberg, Scott; Nori, Harsha; Palangi, Hamid; Ribeiro, Marco Tulio; Zhang, Yi (22 March 2023). "Sparks of Artificial General Intelligence: Early experiments with GPT-4". arXiv:2303.12712 [cs.CL].*
68. *Metz, Cade (1 May 2023). "'The Godfather of A.I.' Leaves Google and Warns of Danger Ahead". The New York Times. ISSN 0362-4331. Retrieved 7 June 2023.*
69. *Nellis, Stephen (2 March 2024). "Nvidia CEO says AI could pass human tests in five years". Reuters.*
70. *Nosta, John (5 January 2024). "The Accelerating Path to Artificial General Intelligence". Psychology Today. Retrieved 30 March 2024.*
71. *Hickey, Alex. "Whole Brain Emulation: A Giant Step for Neuroscience". Tech Brew. Retrieved 8 November 2023.*
72. *Holmgaard Mersh, Amalie (15 September 2023). "Decade-long European research project maps the human brain". euractiv.*
73. Jump up to:[a] [b] *Thornton, Angela (26 June 2023). "How uploading our minds to a computer might become possible". The Conversation. Retrieved 8 November 2023.*
74. *Vicinanza, Domenico (18 December 2023). "A new supercomputer aims to losely mimic the human brain — it could help unlock the secrets of the mind and advance AI". The Conversation. Retrieved 29 March 2024.*
75. *"Artificial General Intelligence – Do[es] the cost outweigh benefits?". 23 August 2021. Retrieved 7 June 2023.*
76. *"How we can Benefit from Advancing Artificial General Intelligence (AGI) – Unite.AI". www.unite.ai. Retrieved 7 June 2023.*
77. Jump up to:[a] [b] [c] *Talty, Jules; Julien, Stephan. "What Will Our Society Look Like When Artificial Intelligence Is Everywhere?". Smithsonian Magazine. Retrieved 7 June 2023.*
78. Jump up to:[a] [b] *Stevenson, Matt (8 October 2015). "Answers to Stephen Hawking's AMA are Here!". Wired. ISSN 1059-1028. Retrieved 8 June 2023.*
79. Jump up to:[a] [b] *Bostrom, Nick (2017). "§ Preferred order of arrival". Superintelligence: paths, dangers, strategies (Reprinted with corrections 2017 ed.). Oxford, United Kingdom; New York, New York, USA: Oxford University Press. ISBN 978-0-19-967811-2.*
80. *Piper, Kelsey (19 November 2018). "How technological progress is making it likelier than ever that humans will destroy ourselves". Vox. Retrieved 8 June 2023.*
81. *Doherty, Ben (17 May 2018). "Climate change an 'existential security risk' to Australia, Senate inquiry says". The Guardian. ISSN 0261-3077. Retrieved 16 July 2023.*

82. *MacAskill, William (2022). What we owe the future. New York, NY: Basic Books. ISBN 978-1-5416-1862-6.*
83. Jump up to:[a] [b] *Ord, Toby (2020). "Chapter 5: Future Risks, Unaligned Artificial Intelligence". The Precipice: Existential Risk and the Future of Humanity. Bloomsbury Publishing. ISBN 978-1-5266-0021-9.*
84. *Al-Sibai, Noor (13 February 2022). "OpenAI Chief Scientist Says Advanced AI May Already Be Conscious". Futurism. Retrieved 24 December 2023.*
85. *Samuelsson, Paul Conrad (2019). "Artificial Consciousness: Our Greatest Ethical Challenge". Philosophy Now. Retrieved 23 December 2023.*
86. *Kateman, Brian (24 July 2023). "AI Should Be Terrified of Humans". TIME. Retrieved 23 December 2023.*
87. *Roose, Kevin (30 May 2023). "A.I. Poses 'Risk of Extinction,' Industry Leaders Warn". The New York Times. ISSN 0362-4331. Retrieved 24 December 2023.*
88. Jump up to:[a] [b] *"Statement on AI Risk". Center for AI Safety. 30 May 2023. Retrieved 8 June 2023.*
89. *"Stephen Hawking: 'Transcendence looks at the implications of artificial intelligence – but are we taking AI seriously enough?'". The Independent (UK). Archived from the original on 25 September 2015. Retrieved 3 December 2014.*
90. *Herger, Mario. "The Gorilla Problem – Enterprise Garage". Retrieved 7 June 2023.*
91. *"The fascinating Facebook debate between Yann LeCun, Stuart Russel and Yoshua Bengio about the risks of strong AI". The fascinating Facebook debate between Yann LeCun, Stuart Russel and Yoshua Bengio about the risks of strong AI (in French). Retrieved 8 June 2023.*
92. *"Will Artificial Intelligence Doom The Human Race Within The Next 100 Years?". HuffPost. 22 August 2014. Retrieved 8 June 2023.*
93. *Sotala, Kaj; Yampolskiy, Roman V. (19 December 2014). "Responses to catastrophic AGI risk: a survey". Physica Scripta.* ***90*** *(1): 018001. doi:10.1088/0031-8949/90/1/018001. ISSN 0031-8949.*
94. *Bostrom, Nick (2014). Superintelligence: Paths, Dangers, Strategies (First ed.). Oxford University Press. ISBN 978-0199678112.*
95. *Chow, Andrew R.; Perrigo, Billy (16 February 2023). "The AI Arms Race Is On. Start Worrying". TIME. Retrieved 24 December 2023.*
96. *Tetlow, Gemma (12 January 2017). "AI arms race risks spiralling out of control, report warns". www.ft.com. Retrieved 24 December 2023.*
97. *Milmo, Dan; Stacey, Kiran (25 September 2023). "Experts disagree over threat posed but artificial intelligence cannot be ignored". The Guardian. ISSN 0261-3077. Retrieved 24 December 2023.*
98. *"Humanity, Security & AI, Oh My! (with Ian Bremmer & Shuman Ghosemajumder)". CAFE. 20 July 2023. Retrieved 15 September 2023.*

99. Hamblin, James (9 May 2014). "But What Would the End of Humanity Mean for Me?". The Atlantic. Archived from the original on 4 June 2014. Retrieved 12 December 2015.

100. Titcomb, James (30 October 2023). "Big Tech is stoking fears over AI, warn scientists". The Telegraph. Retrieved 7 December 2023.

101. "Google Brain founder says big tech is lying about AI extinction danger". Australian Financial Review. 30 October 2023. Retrieved 7 December 2023.

102. "GPTs are GPTs: An early look at the labor market impact potential of large language models". openai.com. Retrieved 7 June 2023.

103. Jump up to:[a] [b] "80% of workers will be exposed to AI. These jobs will be most affected". euronews. 23 March 2023. Retrieved 8 June 2023.

104. Sheffey, Ayelet. "Elon Musk says we need universal basic income because 'in the future, physical work will be a choice'". Business Insider. Retrieved 8 June 2023.

105. UNESCO Science Report: the Race Against Time for Smarter Development. Paris: UNESCO. 11 June 2021. ISBN 978-92-3-100450-6. Archived from the original on 18 June 2022. Retrieved 22 September 2021.

106. Azevedo FA, Carvalho LR, Grinberg LT, Farfel J, et al. (April 2009), "Equal numbers of neuronal and nonneuronal cells make the human brain an isometrically scaled-up primate brain", The Journal of Comparative Neurology, **513** (5): 532–541, doi:10.1002/cne.21974, PMID 19226510, S2CID 5200449, archived from the original on 18 February 2021, retrieved 4 September 2013

107. Halal, William E. "TechCast Article Series: The Automation of Thought" (PDF). Archived from the original (PDF) on 6 June 2013.

108. Kaplan, Andreas (2022). Artificial Intelligence, Business and Civilization: Our Fate Made in Machines. Routledge focus on business and management. New York, NY: Routledge. ISBN 978-1-000-56333-7.

109. Marquis, Pierre; Papini, Odile; Prade, Henri, eds. (2020). A Guided Tour of Artificial Intelligence Research: Volume III: Interfaces and Applications of Artificial Intelligence. Cham: Springer International Publishing. pp. xiii. doi:10.1007/978-3-030-06170-8. ISBN 978-3-030-06169-2.

110. Thomason, James (21 May 2024). "Mojo Rising: The resurgence of AI-first programming languages". VentureBeat. Retrieved 26 May 2024.

111. Wodecki, Ben (5 May 2023). "7 AI Programming Languages You Need to Know". AI Business.

112. Davenport, T; Kalakota, R (June 2019). "The potential for artificial intelligence in healthcare". Future Healthc J. **6** (2): 94–98. doi:10.7861/futurehosp.6-2-94. PMC 6616181. PMID 31363513.

113. Jump up to:[a] [b] Bax, Monique; Thorpe, Jordan; Romanov, Valentin (December 2023). "The future of personalized cardiovascular medicine demands 3D and 4D

*printing, stem cells, and artificial intelligence". Frontiers in Sensors. **4**. doi:10.3389/fsens.2023.1294721. ISSN 2673-5067.*

114. *Jumper, J; Evans, R; Pritzel, A (2021). "Highly accurate protein structure prediction with AlphaFold". Nature. **596** (7873): 583–589. Bibcode:2021Natur.596..583J. doi:10.1038/s41586-021-03819-2. PMC 8371605. PMID 34265844.*
115. *"AI discovers new class of antibiotics to kill drug-resistant bacteria". 20 December 2023.*
116. *"AI speeds up drug design for Parkinson's ten-fold". Cambridge University. 17 April 2024.*
117. *Horne, Robert I.; Andrzejewska, Ewa A.; Alam, Parvez; Brotzakis, Z. Faidon; Srivastava, Ankit; Aubert, Alice; Nowinska, Magdalena; Gregory, Rebecca C.; Staats, Roxine; Possenti, Andrea; Chia, Sean; Sormanni, Pietro; Ghetti, Bernardino; Caughey, Byron; Knowles, Tuomas P. J.; Vendruscolo, Michele (17 April 2024). "Discovery of potent inhibitors of α-synuclein aggregation using structure-based iterative learning". Nature Chemical Biology. **20** (5). Nature: 634–645. doi:10.1038/s41589-024-01580-x. PMC 11062903. PMID 38632492.*
118. *Grant, Eugene F.; Lardner, Rex (25 July 1952). "The Talk of the Town – It". The New Yorker. ISSN 0028-792X. Retrieved 28 January 2024.*
119. *Anderson, Mark Robert (11 May 2017). "Twenty years on from Deep Blue vs Kasparov: how a chess match started the big data revolution". The Conversation. Retrieved 28 January 2024.*
120. *Markoff, John (16 February 2011). "Computer Wins on 'Jeopardy!': Trivial, It's Not". The New York Times. ISSN 0362-4331. Retrieved 28 January 2024.*
121. *Byford, Sam (27 May 2017). "AlphaGo retires from competitive Go after defeating world number one 3–0". The Verge. Retrieved 28 January 2024.*
122. *Brown, Noam; Sandholm, Tuomas (30 August 2019). "Superhuman AI for multiplayer poker". Science. **365** (6456): 885–890. Bibcode:2019Sci...365..885B. doi:10.1126/science.aay2400. ISSN 0036-8075. PMID 31296650.*
123. *"MuZero: Mastering Go, chess, shogi and Atari without rules". Google DeepMind. 23 December 2020. Retrieved 28 January 2024.*
124. *Sample, Ian (30 October 2019). "AI becomes grandmaster in 'fiendishly complex' StarCraft II". The Guardian. ISSN 0261-3077. Retrieved 28 January 2024.*
125. *Wurman, P.R.; Barrett, S.; Kawamoto, K. (2022). "Outracing champion Gran Turismo drivers with deep reinforcement learning". Nature. **602** (7896): 223–228. Bibcode:2022Natur.602..223W. doi:10.1038/s41586-021-04357-7. PMID 35140384.*
126. *Wilkins, Alex (13 March 2024). "Google AI learns to play open-world video games by watching them". New Scientist. Retrieved 21 July 2024.*
127. Matthew Finio & Amanda Downie: IBM Think 2024 Primer, "What is Artificial Intelligence (AI) in Finance?" 8 Dec. 2023

128. Jump up to:[a] [b] *Cao, Longbing (2020). "AI in Finance: A Review". SSRN Electronic Journal. doi:10.2139/ssrn.3647625. ISSN 1556-5068.*
129. M. Nicolas J. Firzli: Pensions Age/European Pensions magazine, "Artificial Intelligence: Ask the Industry" May June 2024 https://videovoice.org/ai-in-finance-innovation-entrepreneurship-vs-over-regulation-with-the-eus-artificial-intelligence-act-wont-work-as-intended/
130. Jump up to:[a] [b] [c] *Congressional Research Service (2019). Artificial Intelligence and National Security (PDF). Washington, DC: Congressional Research Service.*PD-notice
131. Jump up to:[a] [b] *Slyusar, Vadym (2019). "Artificial intelligence as the basis of future control networks". ResearchGate. doi:10.13140/RG.2.2.30247.50087.*
132. *Knight, Will. "The US and 30 Other Nations Agree to Set Guardrails for Military AI". Wired. ISSN 1059-1028. Retrieved 24 January 2024.*
133. *Marcelline, Marco (27 May 2023). "ChatGPT: Most Americans Know About It, But Few Actually Use the AI Chatbot". PCMag. Retrieved 28 January 2024.*
134. *Lu, Donna (31 March 2023). "Misinformation, mistakes and the Pope in a puffer: what rapidly evolving AI can – and can't – do". The Guardian. ISSN 0261-3077. Retrieved 28 January 2024.*
135. *Hurst, Luke (23 May 2023). "How a fake image of a Pentagon explosion shared on Twitter caused a real dip on Wall Street". euronews. Retrieved 28 January 2024.*
136. *Ransbotham, Sam; Kiron, David; Gerbert, Philipp; Reeves, Martin (6 September 2017). "Reshaping Business With Artificial Intelligence". MIT Sloan Management Review. Archived from the original on 13 February 2024.*
137. *Sun, Yuran; Zhao, Xilei; Lovreglio, Ruggiero; Kuligowski, Erica (1 January 2024), Naser, M. Z. (ed.), "8 - AI for large-scale evacuation modeling: promises and challenges", Interpretable Machine Learning for the Analysis, Design, Assessment, and Informed Decision Making for Civil Infrastructure, Woodhead Publishing Series in Civil and Structural Engineering, Woodhead Publishing, pp. 185–204, ISBN 978-0-12-824073-1, retrieved 28 June 2024*
138. *Gomaa, Islam; Adelzadeh, Masoud; Gwynne, Steven; Spencer, Bruce; Ko, Yoon; Bénichou, Noureddine; Ma, Chunyun; Elsagan, Nour; Duong, Dana; Zalok, Ehab; Kinateder, Max (1 November 2021). "A Framework for Intelligent Fire Detection and Evacuation System". Fire Technology.* ***57*** *(6): 3179–3185. doi:10.1007/s10694-021-01157-3. ISSN 1572-8099.*
139. *Zhao, Xilei; Lovreglio, Ruggiero; Nilsson, Daniel (1 May 2020). "Modelling and interpreting pre-evacuation decision-making using machine learning". Automation in Construction.* ***113****: 103140. doi:10.1016/j.autcon.2020.103140. ISSN 0926-5805.*
140. *Kopel, Matthew. "Copyright Services: Fair Use". Cornell University Library. Retrieved 26 April 2024.*
141. *Burgess, Matt. "How to Stop Your Data From Being Used to Train AI". Wired. ISSN 1059-1028. Retrieved 26 April 2024.*

142. *Hammond, George (27 December 2023). "Big Tech is spending more than VC firms on AI startups". Ars Technica. Archived from the original on 10 January 2024.*

143. *Wong, Matteo (24 October 2023). "The Future of AI Is GOMA". The Atlantic. Archived from the original on 5 January 2024.*

144. *"Big tech and the pursuit of AI dominance". The Economist. 26 March 2023. Archived from the original on 29 December 2023.*

145. *Fung, Brian (19 December 2023). "Where the battle to dominate AI may be won". CNN Business. Archived from the original on 13 January 2024.*

146. *Metz, Cade (5 July 2023). "In the Age of A.I., Tech's Little Guys Need Big Friends". The New York Times.*

147. *"Electricity 2024 – Analysis". IEA. 24 January 2024. Retrieved 13 July 2024.*

148. *Calvert, Brian (28 March 2024). "AI already uses as much energy as a small country. It's only the beginning". Vox. New York, NY.*

149. *Halper, Evan; O'Donovan, Caroline (21 June 2024). "AI is exhausting the power grid. Tech firms are seeking a miracle solution". Washington Post.*

150. *Davenport, Carly. "AI Data Centers and the Coming YS Power Demand Surge" (PDF). Goldman Sachs.*

151. *Ryan, Carol (12 April 2024). "Energy-Guzzling AI Is Also the Future of Energy Savings". Wall Street Journal. Dow Jones.*

152. *Hiller, Jennifer (1 July 2024). "Tech Industry Wants to Lock Up Nuclear Power for AI". Wall Street Journal. Dow Jones.*

153. *Rainie, Lee; Keeter, Scott; Perrin, Andrew (22 July 2019). "Trust and Distrust in America". Pew Research Center. Archived from the original on 22 February 2024.*

154. *Ropek, Lucas (21 May 2024). "New Anthropic Research Sheds Light on AI's 'Black Box'". Gizmodo. Retrieved 23 May 2024.*

155. *Buckley, Chris; Mozur, Paul (22 May 2019). "How China Uses High-Tech Surveillance to Subdue Minorities". The New York Times.*

156. *"Security lapse exposed a Chinese smart city surveillance system". 3 May 2019. Archived from the original on 7 March 2021. Retrieved 14 September 2020.*

157. Jump up to:[a] [b] E McGaughey, 'Will Robots Automate Your Job Away? Full Employment, Basic Income, and Economic Democracy' (2022) 51(3) Industrial Law Journal 511–559 Archived 27 May 2023 at the Wayback Machine

158. *Zhou, Viola (11 April 2023). "AI is already taking video game illustrators' jobs in China". Rest of World. Retrieved 17 August 2023.*

159. *Carter, Justin (11 April 2023). "China's game art industry reportedly decimated by growing AI use". Game Developer. Retrieved 17 August 2023.*

160. *Tarnoff, Ben (4 August 2023). "Lessons from Eliza". The Guardian Weekly. pp. 34–39.*

161. *""Godfather of artificial intelligence" talks impact and potential of new AI". CBS News. 25 March 2023. Archived from the original on 28 March 2023. Retrieved 28 March 2023.*

162. Pittis, Don (4 May 2023). "Canadian artificial intelligence leader Geoffrey Hinton piles on fears of computer takeover". CBC.
163. "'50-50 chance' that AI outsmarts humanity, Geoffrey Hinton says - BNN Bloomberg". Bloomberg BNN. 14 June 2024. Retrieved 6 July 2024.
164. Taylor, Josh (7 May 2023). "Rise of artificial intelligence is inevitable but should not be feared, 'father of AI' says". The Guardian. Retrieved 26 May 2023.
165. Colton, Emma (7 May 2023). "'Father of AI' says tech fears misplaced: 'You cannot stop it'". Fox News. Retrieved 26 May 2023.
166. Jones, Hessie (23 May 2023). "Juergen Schmidhuber, Renowned 'Father Of Modern AI,' Says His Life's Work Won't Lead To Dystopia". Forbes. Retrieved 26 May 2023.
167. McMorrow, Ryan (19 December 2023). "Andrew Ng: 'Do we think the world is better off with more or less intelligence?'". Financial Times. Retrieved 30 December 2023.
168. Stewart, Ashley; Melton, Monica. "Hugging Face CEO says he's focused on building a 'sustainable model' for the $4.5 billion open-source-AI startup". Business Insider. Retrieved 14 April 2024.
169. Wiggers, Kyle (9 April 2024). "Google open sources tools to support AI model development". TechCrunch. Retrieved 14 April 2024.
170. Heaven, Will Douglas (12 May 2023). "The open-source AI boom is built on Big Tech's handouts. How long will it last?". MIT Technology Review. Retrieved 14 April 2024.
171. Brodsky, Sascha (19 December 2023). "Mistral AI's New Language Model Aims for Open Source Supremacy". AI Business.
172. Edwards, Benj (22 February 2024). "Stability announces Stable Diffusion 3, a next-gen AI image generator". Ars Technica. Retrieved 14 April 2024.
173. Marshall, Matt (29 January 2024). "How enterprises are using open source LLMs: 16 examples". VentureBeat.
174. Piper, Kelsey (2 February 2024). "Should we make our most powerful AI models open source to all?". Vox. Retrieved 14 April 2024.
175. Alan Turing Institute (2019). "Understanding artificial intelligence ethics and safety" (PDF).
176. Alan Turing Institute (2023). "AI Ethics and Governance in Practice" (PDF).
177. Floridi, Luciano; Cowls, Josh (23 June 2019). "A Unified Framework of Five Principles for AI in Society". Harvard Data Science Review. **1** (1). doi:10.1162/99608f92.8cd550d1. S2CID 198775713.
178. Buruk, Banu; Ekmekci, Perihan Elif; Arda, Berna (1 September 2020). "A critical perspective on guidelines for responsible and trustworthy artificial intelligence". Medicine, Health Care and Philosophy. **23** (3): 387–399. doi:10.1007/s11019-020-09948-1. ISSN 1572-8633. PMID 32236794. S2CID 214766800.

179. *Kamila, Manoj Kumar; Jasrotia, Sahil Singh (1 January 2023). "Ethical issues in the development of artificial intelligence: recognizing the risks". International Journal of Ethics and Systems. ahead-of-print (ahead-of-print). doi:10.1108/IJOES-05-2023-0107. ISSN 2514-9369. S2CID 259614124.*

180. *"AI Safety Institute releases new AI safety evaluations platform". UK Government. 10 May 2024. Retrieved 14 May 2024.*

181. *Russell, Stuart J.; Norvig, Peter. (2021). Artificial Intelligence: A Modern Approach (4th ed.). Hoboken: Pearson. ISBN 978-0134610993. LCCN 20190474.*

182. *Luger, George; Stubblefield, William (2004). Artificial Intelligence: Structures and Strategies for Complex Problem Solving (5th ed.). Benjamin/Cummings. ISBN 978-0-8053-4780-7. Archived from the original on 26 July 2020. Retrieved 17 December 2019.*

183. AI & ML in Fusion, video lecture Archived 2 July 2023 at the Wayback Machine

184. *Alter, Alexandra; Harris, Elizabeth A. (20 September 2023), "Franzen, Grisham and Other Prominent Authors Sue OpenAI", The New York Times*

185. *Altman, Sam; Brockman, Greg; Sutskever, Ilya (22 May 2023). "Governance of Superintelligence". openai.com. Archived from the original on 27 May 2023. Retrieved 27 May 2023.*

186. *"Ask the AI experts: What's driving today's progress in AI?". McKinsey & Company. Archived from the original on 13 April 2018. Retrieved 13 April 2018.*

187. *Barfield, Woodrow; Pagallo, Ugo (2018). Research handbook on the law of artificial intelligence. Cheltenham, UK: Edward Elgar Publishing. ISBN 978-1-78643-904-8. OCLC 1039480085.*

188. *Berlinski, David (2000). The Advent of the Algorithm. Harcourt Books. ISBN 978-0-15-601391-8. OCLC 46890682. Archived from the original on 26 July 2020. Retrieved 22 August 2020.*

189. *Berryhill, Jamie; Heang, Kévin Kok; Clogher, Rob; McBride, Keegan (2019). Hello, World: Artificial Intelligence and its Use in the Public Sector (PDF). Paris: OECD Observatory of Public Sector Innovation. Archived (PDF) from the original on 20 December 2019. Retrieved 9 August 2020.*

190. *Bostrom, Nick (2014). Superintelligence: Paths, Dangers, Strategies. Oxford University Press.*

191. *Bostrom, Nick (2015). "What happens when our computers get smarter than we are?". TED (conference). Archived from the original on 25 July 2020. Retrieved 30 January 2020.*

192. *Brooks, Rodney (10 November 2014). "artificial intelligence is a tool, not a threat". Archived from the original on 12 November 2014.*

193. *Brooks, Rodney (1990). "Elephants Don't Play Chess" (PDF). Robotics and Autonomous Systems.* ***6*** *(1–2): 3–15. CiteSeerX 10.1.1.588.7539. doi:10.1016/S0921-8890(05)80025-9. Archived (PDF) from the original on 9 August 2007.*

194. *Buiten, Miriam C (2019). "Towards Intelligent Regulation of Artificial Intelligence". European Journal of Risk Regulation. **10** (1): 41–59. doi:10.1017/err.2019.8. ISSN 1867-299X.*

195. *Bushwick, Sophie (16 March 2023), "What the New GPT-4 AI Can Do", Scientific American*

196. *Buttazzo, G. (July 2001). "Artificial consciousness: Utopia or real possibility?". Computer. **34** (7): 24–30. doi:10.1109/2.933500.*

197. *DiFeliciantonio, Chase (3 April 2023). "AI has already changed the world. This report shows how". San Francisco Chronicle. Archived from the original on 19 June 2023. Retrieved 19 June 2023.*

198. *Dickson, Ben (2 May 2022). "Machine learning: What is the transformer architecture?". TechTalks. Retrieved 22 November 2023.*

199. *Dockrill, Peter (27 June 2022), "Robots With Flawed AI Make Sexist And Racist Decisions, Experiment Shows", Science Alert, archived from the original on 27 June 2022*

200. *Edwards, Benj (17 May 2023). "Poll: AI poses risk to humanity, according to majority of Americans". Ars Technica. Archived from the original on 19 June 2023. Retrieved 19 June 2023.*

201. *Fox News (2023). "Fox News Poll" (PDF). Fox News. Archived (PDF) from the original on 12 May 2023. Retrieved 19 June 2023.*

202. *Frank, Michael (22 September 2023). "US Leadership in Artificial Intelligence Can Shape the 21st Century Global Order". The Diplomat. Retrieved 8 December 2023. Instead, the United States has developed a new area of dominance that the rest of the world views with a mixture of awe, envy, and resentment: artificial intelligence... From AI models and research to cloud computing and venture capital, U.S. companies, universities, and research labs – and their affiliates in allied countries – appear to have an enormous lead in both developing cutting-edge AI and commercializing it. The value of U.S. venture capital investments in AI start-ups exceeds that of the rest of the world combined.*

203. *Gertner, Jon (18 July 2023). "Wikipedia's Moment of Truth – Can the online encyclopedia help teach A.I. chatbots to get their facts right — without destroying itself in the process? + comment". The New York Times. Archived from the original on 18 July 2023. Retrieved 19 July 2023.*

204. *Goldman, Sharon (14 September 2022). "10 years later, deep learning 'revolution' rages on, say AI pioneers Hinton, LeCun and Li". VentureBeat. Retrieved 8 December 2023.*

205. *Goodfellow, Ian; Bengio, Yoshua; Courville, Aaron (2016), Deep Learning, MIT Press., archived from the original on 16 April 2016, retrieved 12 November 2017*

206. *Goodman, Bryce; Flaxman, Seth (2017). "EU regulations on algorithmic decision-making and a 'right to explanation'". AI Magazine. **38** (3): 50. arXiv:1606.08813. doi:10.1609/aimag.v38i3.2741. S2CID 7373959.*

207. *Government Accountability Office (13 September 2022). Consumer Data: Increasing Use Poses Risks to Privacy. gao.gov (Report).*
208. *Grant, Nico; Hill, Kashmir (22 May 2023). "Google's Photo App Still Can't Find Gorillas. And Neither Can Apple's". The New York Times.*
209. *Goswami, Rohan (5 April 2023). "Here's where the A.I. jobs are". CNBC. Archived from the original on 19 June 2023. Retrieved 19 June 2023.*
210. *Kasperowicz, Peter (1 May 2023). "Regulate AI? GOP much more skeptical than Dems that government can do it right: poll". Fox News. Archived from the original on 19 June 2023. Retrieved 19 June 2023.*
211. *Kissinger, Henry (1 November 2021). "The Challenge of Being Human in the Age of AI". The Wall Street Journal. Archived from the original on 4 November 2021. Retrieved 4 November 2021.*
212. *Kobielus, James (27 November 2019). "GPUs Continue to Dominate the AI Accelerator Market for Now". InformationWeek. Archived from the original on 19 October 2021. Retrieved 11 June 2020.*
213. *Larson, Jeff; Angwin, Julia (23 May 2016). "How We Analyzed the COMPAS Recidivism Algorithm". ProPublica. Archived from the original on 29 April 2019. Retrieved 19 June 2020.*
214. *Laskowski, Nicole (November 2023). "What is Artificial Intelligence and How Does AI Work? TechTarget". Enterprise AI. Retrieved 30 October 2023.*
215. *Lipartito, Kenneth (6 January 2011), The Narrative and the Algorithm: Genres of Credit Reporting from the Nineteenth Century to Today (PDF) (Unpublished manuscript), doi:10.2139/ssrn.1736283, S2CID 166742927, archived (PDF) from the original on 9 October 2022*
216. *McCarthy, John; Minsky, Marvin; Rochester, Nathan; Shannon, Claude (1955). "A Proposal for the Dartmouth Summer Research Project on Artificial Intelligence". Archived from the original on 26 August 2007. Retrieved 30 August 2007.*
217. *McGaughey, E (2022), Will Robots Automate Your Job Away? Full Employment, Basic Income, and Economic Democracy, p. 51(3) Industrial Law Journal 511–559, doi:10.2139/ssrn.3044448, S2CID 219336439, SSRN 3044448, archived from the original on 31 January 2021, retrieved 27 May 2023*
218. *Poria, Soujanya; Cambria, Erik; Bajpai, Rajiv; Hussain, Amir (September 2017). "A review of affective computing: From unimodal analysis to multimodal fusion". Information Fusion. 37: 98–125. doi:10.1016/j.inffus.2017.02.003. hdl:1893/25490. S2CID 205433041. Archived from the original on 23 March 2023. Retrieved 27 April 2021.*
219. *Reisner, Alex (19 August 2023), "Revealed: The Authors Whose Pirated Books are Powering Generative AI", The Atlantic*
220. *Rose, Steve (11 July 2023). "AI Utopia or dystopia?". The Guardian Weekly. pp. 42–43.Schmidhuber, Jürgen (2022). "Annotated History of Modern AI and Deep Learning".*

221. *Smith, Craig S. (15 March 2023). "ChatGPT-4 Creator Ilya Sutskever on AI Hallucinations and AI Democracy". Forbes. Retrieved 25 December 2023.*

222. *Smoliar, Stephen W.; Zhang, HongJiang (1994). "Content based video indexing and retrieval". IEEE MultiMedia. **1** (2): 62–72. doi:10.1109/93.311653. S2CID 32710913.*

223. *Stanford University (2023). "Artificial Intelligence Index Report 2023/Chapter 6: Policy and Governance" (PDF). AI Index. Archived (PDF) from the original on 19 June 2023. Retrieved 19 June 2023.*

224. *Tao, Jianhua; Tan, Tieniu (2005). Affective Computing and Intelligent Interaction. Affective Computing: A Review. Lecture Notes in Computer Science. Vol. 3784. Springer. pp. 981–995. doi:10.1007/11573548. ISBN 978-3-540-29621-8.*

225. *Taylor, Josh; Hern, Alex (2 May 2023). "'Godfather of AI' Geoffrey Hinton quits Google and warns over dangers of misinformation". The Guardian.*

226. *Thro, Ellen (1993). Robotics: The Marriage of Computers and Machines. New York: Facts on File. ISBN 978-0-8160-2628-9. Archived from the original on 26 July 2020. Retrieved 22 August 2020.*

227. *Toews, Rob (3 September 2023). "Transformers Revolutionized AI. What Will Replace Them?". Forbes. Retrieved 8 December 2023.*

228. *UNESCO Science Report: the Race Against Time for Smarter Development. Paris: UNESCO. 2021. ISBN 978-92-3-100450-6. Archived from the original on 18 June 2022. Retrieved 18 September 2021.*

229. *Urbina, Fabio; Lentzos, Filippa; Invernizzi, Cédric; Ekins, Sean (7 March 2022). "Dual use of artificial-intelligence-powered drug discovery". Nature Machine Intelligence. **4** (3): 189–191. doi:10.1038/s42256-022-00465-9. PMC 9544280. PMID 36211133. S2CID 247302391.*

230. *Valance, Christ (30 May 2023). "Artificial intelligence could lead to extinction, experts warn". BBC News. Archived from the original on 17 June 2023. Retrieved 18 June 2023.*

231. *Verma, Yugesh (25 December 2021). "A Complete Guide to SHAP – SHAPley Additive exPlanations for Practitioners". Analytics India Magazine. Retrieved 25 November 2023.*

232. *Vincent, James (7 November 2019). "OpenAI has published the text-generating AI it said was too dangerous to share". The Verge. Archived from the original on 11 June 2020. Retrieved 11 June 2020.*

233. *Vincent, James (15 November 2022). "The scary truth about AI copyright is nobody knows what will happen next". The Verge. Archived from the original on 19 June 2023. Retrieved 19 June 2023.*

234. *Vincent, James (3 April 2023). "AI is entering an era of corporate control". The Verge. Archived from the original on 19 June 2023. Retrieved 19 June 2023.*

235. *Vinge, Vernor (1993). "The Coming Technological Singularity: How to Survive in the Post-Human Era". Vision 21: Interdisciplinary Science and Engineering in the*

Era of Cyberspace: 11. Bibcode:1993vise.nasa...11V. Archived from the original on 1 January 2007. Retrieved 14 November 2011.

236. *Waddell, Kaveh (2018). "Chatbots Have Entered the Uncanny Valley". The Atlantic. Archived from the original on 24 April 2018. Retrieved 24 April 2018.*

237. *"What is 'fuzzy logic'? Are there computers that are inherently fuzzy and do not apply the usual binary logic?". Scientific American. 21 October 1999. Archived from the original on 6 May 2018. Retrieved 5 May 2018.*

238. *Williams, Rhiannon (28 June 2023), "Humans may be more likely to believe disinformation generated by AI", MIT Technology Review*

239. *Wirtz, Bernd W.; Weyerer, Jan C.; Geyer, Carolin (24 July 2018). "Artificial Intelligence and the Public Sector – Applications and Challenges". International Journal of Public Administration.* ***42*** *(7): 596–615. doi:10.1080/01900692.2018.1498103. ISSN 0190-0692. S2CID 158829602. Archived from the original on 18 August 2020. Retrieved 22 August 2020.*

240. *Wong, Matteo (19 May 2023), "ChatGPT Is Already Obsolete", The Atlantic*

241. *Yudkowsky, E (2008), "Artificial Intelligence as a Positive and Negative Factor in Global Risk" (PDF), Global Catastrophic Risks, Oxford University Press, 2008, Bibcode:2008gcr..book..303Y, archived (PDF) from the original on 19 October 2013, retrieved 24 September 2021*

242. Ashish Vaswani, Noam Shazeer, Niki Parmar et al. "Attention is all you need." Advances in neural information processing systems 30 (2017). Seminal paper on transformers.

243. Autor, David H., "Why Are There Still So Many Jobs? The History and Future of Workplace Automation" (2015) 29(3) *Journal of Economic Perspectives* 3.

244. Cukier, Kenneth, "Ready for Robots? How to Think about the Future of AI", *Foreign Affairs*, vol. 98, no. 4 (July/August 2019), pp. 192–98. George Dyson, historian of computing, writes (in what might be called "Dyson's Law") that "Any system simple enough to be understandable will not be complicated enough to behave intelligently, while any system complicated enough to behave intelligently will be too complicated to understand." (p. 197.) Computer scientist Alex Pentland writes: "Current AI machine-learning algorithms are, at their core, dead simple stupid. They work, but they work by brute force." (p. 198.)

245. Gertner, Jon. (2023) "Wikipedia's Moment of Truth: Can the online encyclopedia help teach A.I. chatbots to get their facts right — without destroying itself in the process?" *New York Times Magazine* (July 18, 2023) online

246. Gleick, James, "The Fate of Free Will" (review of Kevin J. Mitchell, *Free Agents: How Evolution Gave Us Free Will*, Princeton University Press, 2023, 333 pp.), *The New York Review of Books*, vol. LXXI, no. 1 (18 January 2024), pp. 27–28, 30. "Agency is what distinguishes us from machines. For biological creatures, reason and purpose come from acting in the world and experiencing the

consequences. Artificial intelligences – disembodied, strangers to blood, sweat, and tears – have no occasion for that." (p. 30.)

247. Hughes-Castleberry, Kenna, "A Murder Mystery Puzzle: The literary puzzle *Cain's Jawbone*, which has stumped humans for decades, reveals the limitations of natural-language-processing algorithms", *Scientific American*, vol. 329, no. 4 (November 2023), pp. 81–82. "This murder mystery competition has revealed that although NLP (natural-language processing) models are capable of incredible feats, their abilities are very much limited by the amount of context they receive. This [...] could cause [difficulties] for researchers who hope to use them to do things such as analyze ancient languages. In some cases, there are few historical records on long-gone civilizations to serve as training data for such a purpose." (p. 82.)

248. Immerwahr, Daniel, "Your Lying Eyes: People now use A.I. to generate fake videos indistinguishable from real ones. How much does it matter?", *The New Yorker*, 20 November 2023, pp. 54–59. "If by 'deepfakes' we mean realistic videos produced using artificial intelligence that actually deceive people, then they barely exist. The fakes aren't deep, and the deeps aren't fake. [...] A.I.-generated videos are not, in general, operating in our media as counterfeited evidence. Their role better resembles that of cartoons, especially smutty ones." (p. 59.)

249. *Jumper, John; Evans, Richard; Pritzel, Alexander; et al. (26 August 2021). "Highly accurate protein structure prediction with AlphaFold". Nature. **596** (7873): 583–589. Bibcode:2021Natur.596..583J. doi:10.1038/s41586-021-03819-2. PMC 8371605. PMID 34265844. S2CID 235959867.*

250. *LeCun, Yann; Bengio, Yoshua; Hinton, Geoffrey (28 May 2015). "Deep learning". Nature. **521** (7553): 436–444. Bibcode:2015Natur.521..436L. doi:10.1038/nature14539. PMID 26017442. S2CID 3074096. Archived from the original on 5 June 2023. Retrieved 19 June 2023.*

251. Marcus, Gary, "Artificial Confidence: Even the newest, buzziest systems of artificial general intelligence are stymmied by the same old problems", *Scientific American*, vol. 327, no. 4 (October 2022), pp. 42–45.

252. *Mitchell, Melanie (2019). Artificial intelligence: a guide for thinking humans. New York: Farrar, Straus and Giroux. ISBN 9780374257835.*

253. *Mnih, Volodymyr; Kavukcuoglu, Koray; Silver, David; et al. (26 February 2015). "Human-level control through deep reinforcement learning". Nature. **518** (7540): 529–533. Bibcode:2015Natur.518..529M. doi:10.1038/nature14236. PMID 25719670. S2CID 205242740. Archived from the original on 19 June 2023. Retrieved 19 June 2023.* Introduced DQN, which produced human-level performance on some Atari games.

254. Press, Eyal, "In Front of Their Faces: Does facial-recognition technology lead police to ignore contradictory evidence?", *The New Yorker*, 20 November 2023, pp. 20–26.
255. Roivainen, Eka, "AI's IQ: ChatGPT aced a [standard intelligence] test but showed that intelligence cannot be measured by IQ alone", *Scientific American*, vol. 329, no. 1 (July/August 2023), p. 7. "Despite its high IQ, ChatGPT fails at tasks that require real humanlike reasoning or an understanding of the physical and social world.... ChatGPT seemed unable to reason logically and tried to rely on its vast database of... facts derived from online texts."
256. *Serenko, Alexander; Michael Dohan (2011). "Comparing the expert survey and citation impact journal ranking methods: Example from the field of Artificial Intelligence" (PDF). Journal of Informetrics.* ***5*** *(4): 629–49. doi:10.1016/j.joi.2011.06.002. Archived (PDF) from the original on 4 October 2013. Retrieved 12 September 2013.*
257. *Silver, David; Huang, Aja; Maddison, Chris J.; et al. (28 January 2016). "Mastering the game of Go with deep neural networks and tree search". Nature.* ***529*** *(7587): 484–489. Bibcode:2016Natur.529..484S. doi:10.1038/nature16961. PMID 26819042. S2CID 515925. Archived from the original on 18 June 2023. Retrieved 19 June 2023.*
258. *White Paper: On Artificial Intelligence – A European approach to excellence and trust (PDF). Brussels: European Commission. 2020. Archived (PDF) from the original on 20 February 2020. Retrieved 20 February 2020.*